Nutrition in Immune Balance (NIMBAL) Therapy
Using Diet to Treat Inflammatory Bowel Disease

Nutrition in Immune Balance (NIMBAL) Therapy

Using Diet to Treat Inflammatory Bowel Disease

David L. Suskind, MD

Professor of Pediatrics,
University of Washington

Division of Gastroenterology, Hepatology and Nutrition,
Seattle Children's Hospital

Published by Nimbal Publishing, LLC.

To order additional copies of this book, inquire about discounts, or find out more information, please visit **www.nimbal.org**.

First Edition
ISBN: 978-0-692-43099-6
Library of Congress Control Number: 1-2305607441

Printed in the USA by BookPrinting.com.
Cover and book design by Mi Ae Lipe, What Now Design, LLC.

Front cover photo: Olha Afanasieva, Dreamstime.com.
Back cover photo: Elena Elisseeva, Dreamstime.com.
Photos throughout book are from Dreamstime.com, iStock.com, and Shutterstock.com unless otherwise specified.
Photos on pages 1, 18, 30, 37, 41, 48, 81, and 86 by David L. Suskind.
Photos on pages 68, 74, and 87 by Tali Guday.

This book is designed to assist patients, parents, and healthcare practitioners deal with dietary management of IBD. It is intended to be a reference only and not an in-depth review of either nutritional or medical issues that occur in inflammatory bowel disease. This book is an educational resource only and none of its content is meant to be standard of care.

To the loves in my life—Rebecca, Elias, and Sadie—
and the foundation from which I grew—Mom and Dad.

Contents

The Specific Carbohydrate Diet: What It Is and If It's Right for You

Getting on the SCD and Sticking with It

How to SCD Everyday

Preparing SCD Food

SCD Recipes

How to Know If the SCD Is Working for You

Alternatives to SCD

Frequently Asked Questions

The Future of SCD

Preface

Each year tens of thousands of individuals are diagnosed with inflammatory bowel disease, or IBD, in the form of ulcerative colitis and Crohn's disease. Currently, there are an estimated 1.3 million individuals in the United States with IBD. The incidence of IBD continues to rise in America, and a major culprit is our food environment. Our diets directly affect our fecal microbiomes and the hundred trillion bacteria that naturally reside in our digestive tracts and bowels. With IBD, what we eat can cause these bacteria to get out of balance and thus trigger our immune systems to attack the bowels.

Poor nutrition also profoundly impacts an individual's overall well-being, ravaging not only our energy but also profoundly affecting every organ system within our bodies. But in spite of their obvious importance, nutrition and diet are often overlooked in the worlds of medicine and science.

This book is the realization of a long-held dream by me and many at Seattle Children's Hospital to support patients and families interested in pursuing nutritional and dietary management for IBD. Nutrition in Immune Balance (NIMBAL) therapy is a standardized method to incorporate dietary therapy into the current medical paradigm. This book is only a first step in developing a standard approach to dietary intervention in IBD; much more research and knowledge still need to be gathered to optimize dietary approaches for IBD patients.

As with every aspect of medicine, diets often need to be individualized for each person and situation. This book is designed to assist patients with IBD, their families, and their healthcare providers on how to begin approaching and using dietary interventions and treatment.

I would like to recognize the many people who have helped to make this book possible through their continued support, content, and review.

David L. Suskind, MD
Seattle, Washington
May 5, 2015

Acknowledgments

Much appreciation to Tali, Shai, and Gil Guday for their strength, insight, and commitment to using diet as a treatment for IBD. Also major thanks to Mi Ae Lipe and Lisa Gordanier for their astounding abilities, diligence, and dedication to this project, and to Rebecca Davis for her expertise in wordsmithing.

Appreciation also to Travis Bettinson and all of the SCD families for their many delicious recipes.

And finally to the most amazing pediatric IBD team at Seattle Children's Hospital—Ghassan Wahbeh, Kim Braly, Nila Williamson, Teresa Wachs, Dale Lee, Matt Giefer, Chinonyelum Obih, Heather Nielson, Jani Klein, and the wonderful Heidi Zogorski.

Disclaimer

This book is designed to assist patients, parents, and healthcare practitioners with the dietary management of inflammatory bowel disease (IBD). It is intended to be a reference only and not an in-depth review of either nutritional or medical issues that occur in IBD. This book is an educational resource only, and none of its content is meant to be a standard of care. The author would like to acknowledge Seattle Children's Hospital for its continued commitment to the importance of nutrition in pediatric health.

A Note to Our Readers

This book has been written for both pediatric patients with IBD and their parents, and we freely refer to both throughout the book, sometimes going back and forth within a chapter. We also prefer to not refer to an individual child as an awkward "he or she"; instead, we often switch to the generic plural pronoun "they" or "their" within a sentence. Or we may refer to a child as "he" in one paragraph, and "she" in another. With this language, in no way do we intend any preference of one gender over the other.

Inflammatory Bowel Disease: An Introduction

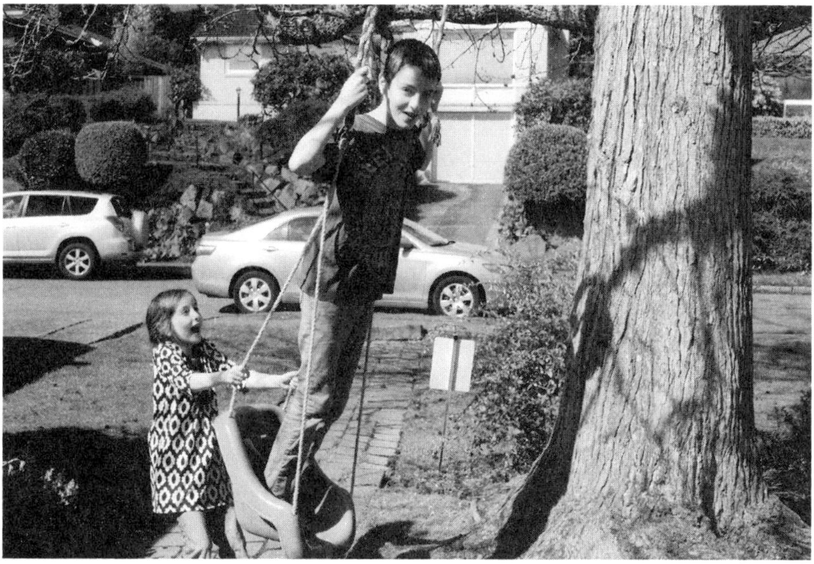

What is inflammatory bowel disease (IBD)?

Our bodies have many systems that keep us healthy and living. One of these is our immune system, which helps prevent as well as fight off infection, protecting us from serious illness. It keeps us from getting simple infections like the kind you can get by cutting yourself, and it protects us from potentially life-threatening infections such as pneumonia and meningitis. It doesn't always work perfectly, but it goes a long way in keeping us safe from harmful events and illnesses.

Unfortunately, sometimes the immune system forgets its role. Instead of protecting us, it starts to attack us. This is called "immune dysregulation."

Inflammatory bowel disease is one example of that.

Why does this occur?

We don't know with perfect certainty why someone gets IBD, but what we do know is that our genes play an important role in the development of the disease. Some of us have a genetic predisposition to IBD, meaning that the genes that make up our immune system lead our immune systems to more likely attack our bowels. IBD is associated with more than 160 different genetic changes, and most of those are related to the immune system. But genes by themselves don't cause IBD. For many millennium, our genes have been the same or very similar to our ancestors. However, our ancestors did not have nearly the same incidence of IBD as we see today.

Additionally, studies show that the incidence of IBD rises significantly depending on where you live. For example, if you are born in India and move to the United Kingdom as an adult, the chances of developing IBD are low, similar to people who stay living in India. But if you are the offspring of that person and thus were born in the UK and grew up in the UK, then your chances of developing IBD become much higher—equal to that of the families around you. Both of these facts point to the assumption that there may be an ecological or environmental trigger for IBD. Although scientists are still searching for the key trigger, mounting evidence indicates that it may be fecal dysbiosis, or "bad bacteria" in our intestines. More about this later.

A couple of important facts about IBD

We know that immune dysregulation disorders such as inflammatory bowel disease are on the rise. This has been true for several decades.

We also know that these disorders are much more common in industrialized countries than in less economically developed countries. In the United States alone, over 1.3 million people suffer from IBD. The most susceptible population? Young adults and teens. At least 100,000 children under the age of 18 in the United States have been diagnosed with IBD.

What are the types of inflammatory bowel disease?

Two main subtypes of IBD exist: Crohn's disease and ulcerative colitis. Both are characterized by an attack on the bowels by the immune system, causing the harmful inflammation in IBD. The two subtypes differ in where the attack occurs, how the patient is affected, the way each progresses clinically, and how the disease looks to the healthcare provider.

Crohn's disease

In Crohn's disease, inflammation can occur anywhere from the mouth to the anus. Inflammation can result in stricturing (narrowing of the bowels) or the formation of abscesses and fistulas, which are abnormal connections between the bowels and the skin, bowel, or organ. Crohn's disease is usually described as being "patchy," involving just one part or many parts of the bowels.

With Crohn's, people can experience a variety of symptoms, which usually depend upon what part of the bowels is affected and how much inflammation is present. Some individuals may have recurrent oral ulcers that can make eating uncomfortable.

If the stomach or duodenum (first part of the small intestines) is affected, people can have pain in their upper abdomen. The small intestine (which is made up of three parts—the duodenum, jejunum, and ileum) is the longest part of the intestines but has the smallest diameter (thus its name "small intestines"). Its main job is to absorb nutrients. When this is affected, people can develop significant abdominal pain as well as nutritional deficiencies and weight loss. The small intestine is affected in approximately two-thirds of people with Crohn's disease.

The colon is the last part of the intestines before the stool leaves the body. It is called the large intestine because its diameter is bigger than that of the small intestine. One of the colon's many jobs is to absorb excess water in the stool. When the colon gets irritated or inflamed, people usually develop diarrhea and cramping with bowel movements. If the rectum (the last part of the colon) gets irritated, it sends messages to the brain that there is still stool within it.

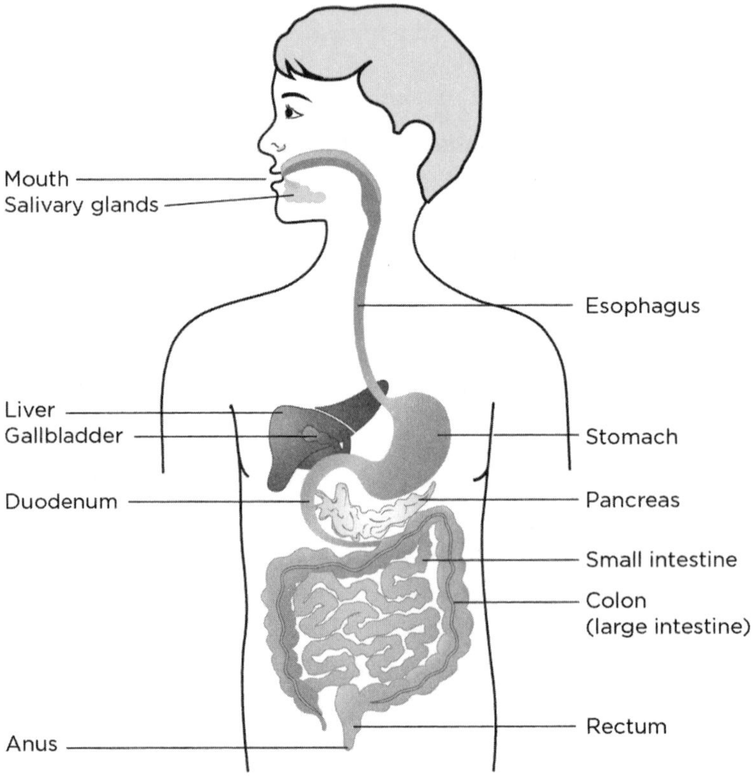

Therefore, patients often complain about the need to go the bathroom without anything or just a small amount of stool coming out. This is called "tenesmus." When the colon is affected, a fair amount of blood can sometimes leak into the stool; therefore colonic disease is characterized by bloody diarrhea.

While medicines are effective in treating it, active Crohn's disease also carries a high likelihood of the need for surgery within five years of diagnosis. This surgery will not, unfortunately, cure the patient of his or her Crohn's.

Ulcerative colitis (UC)

In ulcerative colitis (UC), inflammation is present within the colon (large intestines) and is contiguous, meaning that it starts at the rectum and continues without interruption through the colon. For some, only a small part of the colon is affected. If the inflammation is in the rectum, it is called "proctitis." For others, the entire colon can be involved. This is called "pancolitis." Symptoms of ulcerative colitis are the same as if someone had Crohn's colitis, with symptoms dependent on the degree and extent of disease. Unlike Crohn's disease, if you have surgery to remove the colon to treat the UC, the disease can be cured.

Other IBD manifestations and factors

While we talk mostly about two types of IBD—Crohn's and ulcerative colitis—in truth, the term represents many different types of bowel disease, and each individual is unique in their presentation, response to medication, and journey. With that said, there are commonalities for individuals with IBD, and long-term observation has taught us a lot about the disease. Our ever-expanding technology gives us more tools to determine genetic and environmental influences on diseases and how they express themselves in each of us.

For example, we know that if you smoke and have Crohn's, your disease is far more difficult to treat. If you are a smoker and have UC and you stop smoking, there is a higher likelihood that you will have a flare-up of your symptoms. (Of course, it is best to stop smoking to improve overall health.)

We also know that IBD is more common in the northern hemisphere than in the southern one. If you have the genetic abnormality NOD2, your disease is more likely to be in the ileum, or last section of the small intestine. Younger children usually present with more aggressive UC than their adult counterparts, and more often than not, pediatric UC affects the entire colon.

Most importantly, no matter how much we know about epidemiology and science, IBD is highly personal and specific to each individual. One person's experience with ulcerative colitis or Crohn's is not necessarily identical to another's.

What happens now?

The more you know, the easier it will be.

A diagnosis of inflammatory bowel disease can be overwhelming. It can be a shock, and it can be depressing. But the first thing to say to yourself is, "We have a problem, we are going to handle it, and we are going to find a way to solve it the best way we can." Being proactive, believe it or not, is halfway to a cure.

One of the most pressing questions you'll have is, *how exactly will this affect my child's life?*

There are a few answers. A good place to begin is with your healthcare provider. Ask the questions you need answers to (writing them down beforehand helps). If necessary, be self-assured enough to say, "I really don't understand what you're saying," or "Perhaps you didn't really understand what I was asking you." The more honest you can be, the clearer you are, and the more likely you'll get the answers you need.

Read—a lot. Find out from those who have gone through this before which books and resources they found most helpful. Here, I would caution about the Internet. I have found more misleading than factual information online, and this sometimes leads newly diagnosed families to panic. Don't panic—join support groups instead. Sometimes reassurance comes not just from what you hear in these groups, but from being with others who are going through the same experience—because while you'll learn from them, they will also learn from you.

It is impossible to become an expert overnight

Over time, with the support of friends, family, your medical healthcare practitioner, and especially others with inflammatory bowel disease, you will understand the disease, you will be able to help yourself and your child, and both of you will live a healthy, happy life, even while living with IBD.

Let me tell you my story

Right after my twelfth birthday, I was diagnosed with Type 1 diabetes. My family was overseas at the time. The first indication that something was amiss was when I got so angry waiting for dinner that I kicked the tires of somebody else's car. Because I was always the nicest, most polite child in our family (well … that's the way I remember me, no matter what my brother and sisters say!), this was quite unexpected behavior from me.

After watching me attack the defenseless tires, my mother's first thought was, "Ah, the beginnings of puberty!" Not so. Two days later, a friend who was a doctor heard about what happened and was also told that I was constantly complaining of being thirsty. He said, "I think we ought to do a urine test." My mother said she didn't think much about it, even when the friend called back and said I was "throwing ketones," an indication of diabetes. To her, "diabetes" was just a word with little meaning.

It was after she understood the profound change it would mean for me—and its lifelong effects—that she said she crumbled inside. I never really knew it, of course. But the adjustment for me and my family was major. My family needed to learn what diabetes really meant for me and for them as my family. Would it affect me psychologically? Would it make me feel different, or change my personality? Could I continue to learn? Would I go blind? Because they loved me, they were concerned for what the future held for me.

Now I am going to tell you something you may have a hard time believing, but it is absolutely true: The effect that diabetes has had on my life has been a positive one. How can I truthfully say that? It is because it has shaped the way I live and experience my life. And, I really love my life.

This is not to say I didn't have bad days or that I wouldn't be ecstatic if a cure was found. But because my parents, my family, and I dealt with diabetes not as a hindrance but as just another aspect of my life I needed to work with, I learned that all obstacles life throws at you, big and small, have to be handled in the most positive way possible. I live with my disease, I try to make it as unobtrusive as possible, and most importantly, I don't let it define me.

Let me repeat that: I have diabetes, but I also have a sense of humor, the ability to grow (really good) plums in my backyard, to play soccer with my children, and to enjoy my wife's really great cooking. All of this, including diabetes, is what makes me me.

This is true for all of us with chronic diseases. We have them, we manage them, and they are a part of our lives. But—and this is an important but—they are not us. They are only one aspect of us. My advice to parents of children with IBD is to make sure your child is encouraged to live fully in all the realms of their life so that, as an adult, the world is full of opportunity and stimulation, not obstacles and disease.

What can a parent do?

The most important thing a parent can do is to give a child support, reassurance, guidance, and love. And, when it is you as the parent who needs help, reach out to those who can give you that same support, reassurance, guidance, and love in turn. Supportive friends, family, and community can make all the difference.

Make sure that your child receives the best healthcare available. Speak up when you have questions, especially when those questions come from the child who is learning about their disease. I'm a big fan of the summer camps and the many wonderful programs for young adults and children with IBD, including those put on by the Crohn's and Colitis Foundation of America (CCFA). These can help them realize that they are not alone and that a like-minded community is there to support them. Knowing that you are not alone is a great boost to the brain and self-esteem!

Knowing What the Doctors Know: Genetics and Environment

The role of gene abnormalities

A genetic component does contribute to the development of inflammatory bowel disease. Over 160 genetic risk markers, or genes that can lead to IBD, have already been identified.

The most common gene abnormality found in Crohn's is the NOD2 gene. About 15% of individuals with Crohn's have it. This gene, as well as many others, are involved in regulating what goes on in the lining of the intestine. Their role is to protect that lining—and therefore the person—from a bacterial invasion.

Bacterial invasion?! Sounds like war, right? And, in fact, for the person with IBD, that's just what it is. These genes regulate the immune system, acting as a defense against intestinal bacterial invasion and making sure that what takes place in the intestine stays there.

That said, the genetic abnormalities do not by themselves cause inflammatory bowel disease; individuals can have them and still not develop IBD. A good example of this can be seen in identical twins, who share exactly the same genetic makeup. Yet, the chance of identical twins both having IBD is less than 50%. If genes alone caused IBD, it would occur in 100% of identical twins.

That means, of course, that we have to look for a second factor, something that triggers the disease process in people who are genetically susceptible. And that's exactly what we are trying to figure out.

The world of gut bacteria and fecal dysbiosis

Fecal dysbiosis. Sounds awful, right? Well, it *is* awful, and it seems to be the basic cause of IBD. What is it, exactly? Well, *dysbiosis* literally means "bad bacteria." In us, it means a kind of bacterial imbalance. And, considering just *how many* bacteria are in our intestines, a sudden crowd of mean, belligerent, bully bacteria means, as you might well guess, trouble.

But time out first for a quick thank you to Dutch scientist Antonie van Leeuwenhoek. In 1688, van Leeuwenhoek started building a microscope strong enough to see tiny, tiny cells. He called them "animalcules," and today we call them "microorganisms."

Because of him, we know that lots more bacteria live within our intestines then there are actual cells that make up our entire body. As van Leeuwenhoek said to the Royal British society, "The people living in our United Netherlands [where he was originally from] are not as many as the living animals that I carry in my mouth." At the time, however, even he did not realize how right he was. There are over 100 *trillion* microorganisms in our bowels. One hundred trillion! This is 10 *times* more than the number of human cells in the body!

To make this picture even clearer, the human gut alone contains about three pounds of bacteria. Their collective genome encodes around three million different genes. That's more than 100 times our own. Our bacteria live within us in large numbers and are very active!

Why do we have so many of these guys? When we think of bacteria, we automatically tend to regard them as something bad. However, these bacteria have been a part of us for as long as humans have been around. As we've evolved, they've evolved with us. Most of the time these bacteria help us. They break down indigestible carbohydrates and produce small-chain fatty acids, which our colons use as nutrients. They produce essential vitamins important for our overall health. They also coat our intestines, decreasing the possibility that bad bacteria can take over and infect our bowels.

If we think of our intestines as a diverse community within us, we call that particular population a microbiome. This refers to all of the microorganisms that live in our bodies: the good bacteria ("symbiotic" bacteria), the neither-good-nor-bad bacteria (the "commensal" bacteria), and finally, the not-so-good disease-causing bacteria ("pathogenic" bacteria).

Like individuals living in a community (such as the people living in your city or town), these microorganisms—our "microbiota"—change. Some move out, new ones move in, and all of them are adapting in response to changes in their environment. While the people in a city may fluctuate depending on economics, schooling, and other resources, the bacteria in your bowels change depending on the food you eat, the activities you do, and the medications you take. And just like people, bacteria also adapt to the environment that they're in.

The first year of our lives: What's growing in our intestines?

Let's take it from the very beginning. When you were growing in your mother's womb, your environment was a sterile one. You had no bacteria in your bowels. But as soon as you were born and left that nice, peaceful, sterile environment, everything changed. In fact, as we are being born, we are given some of our mother's bacteria.

The variety and types of bacteria you receive as a baby depends on many factors. Your bacteria will be different depending on whether you were born by Caesarean section versus vaginally. They will also be different whether you were breast-fed or bottle-fed. These variations can create profound differences in your body, including the amount of infection and colic you may have had as a baby. If you were given antibiotics during your first year of life, your gut bacteria can and most likely will be altered. In fact, the use of antibiotics during this early period of growth is now linked with a higher chance of developing inflammatory bowel disease.

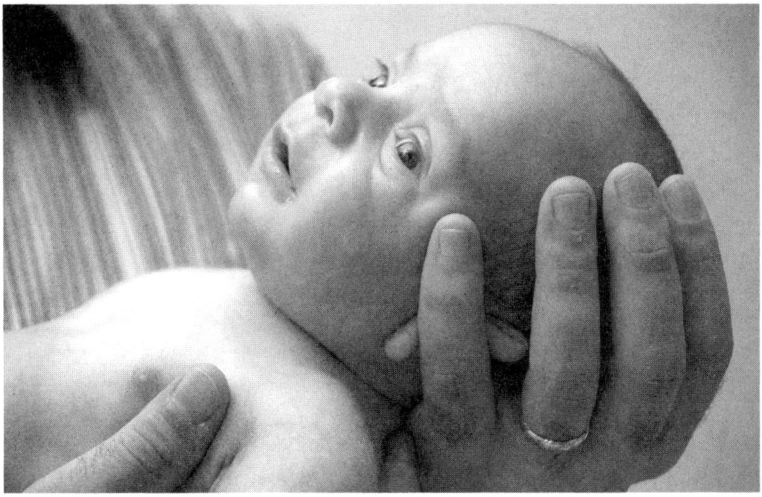

In the meantime, what's growing? Lots and lots of bacteria. This happens because the intestines start to mature, and as a baby is introduced to more varied foods, more bacteria are encouraged to grow in turn. By a baby's first birthday, the bacteria within an infant's bowel is starting to resemble what we see in the adult microbiota, but it is still developing and it isn't until 3 to 4 years of age that a more mature microbiota is formed. As we mentioned before, the sheer numbers we carry within us as adults are staggering—more than 100 trillion bacteria with more than 1,000 different species! This is an important part of growing and developing a child's immune system, so that it can learn which bacteria are pathologic (bad) and which are good, or at least harmless.

Do these bacteria play a role in developing IBD?

The fecal microbiome is extremely complex. Our current knowledge only scrapes at the surface of what is to be learned. Currently we think that there are both good and bad bacteria, plus a large number that may be neither beneficial nor harmful. All of these bacteria interplay with the immune system in ways yet to be understood that may develop into IBD.

In animal studies, the fecal microbiota appears to be critical for maintaining intestinal well-being. In animal models, certain genetically modified animals develop colitis only in the presence of bacteria. These animals will not develop colitis without bacteria in their gut. In human studies, individuals with inflammatory bowel disease have much less bacterial diversity. The mechanism by which this contributes to IBD is not well defined, but it could be that this decreased diversity may allow invasive bacterial species to increase, coupled with decreased protective bacteria. This could result in inappropriate immune cell activation and loss of immunologic tolerance. But we still have much to learn.

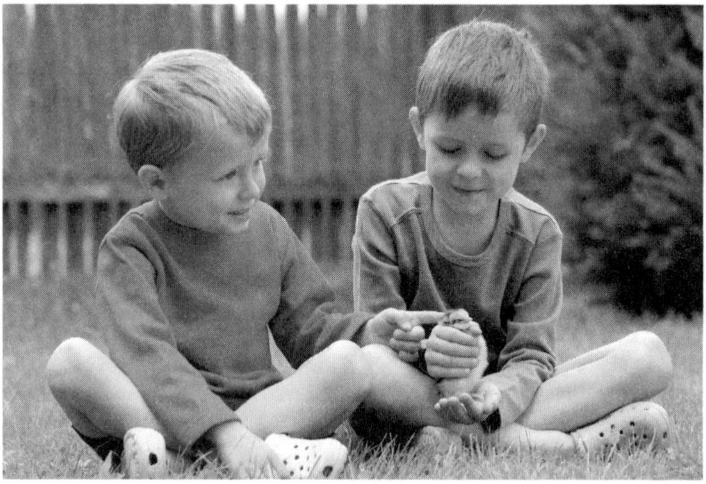

For doctors, however, the pressing question remains: Why has IBD become so common? Our genes make us who we are, often determining whether we will be sick or healthy. They have been reproduced in humans for thousands of years. Over time, the bacteria within our bowels have adapted to us as well, meaning that our bodies have not only gotten used to them but use them—even depend on them—for our overall well-being.

So why now are the bacteria of many people making them sick and allowing IBD to become such a common disorder of the bowels?

The answer is not totally clear, but if we believe that fecal dysbiosis—bad bacteria within our bowels—is making us sick, why have those bacteria that have adapted to us over the millennia changed? Many possibilities abound. However, two key culprits are most likely to blame: antibiotic use and dietary changes.

The role of modern antibiotics

While we're not going to go into extensive detail regarding the impact of antibiotics on the development of IBD in this book, it's important to recognize that antibiotics have played a critical and positive role in human health history, saving many lives.

However, what we are discussing now is the current overuse of antibiotics and its negative effects on our health. The most obvious is the bacterial resistance we see and read about in the media. What does this mean? When antibiotics were first prescribed to knock out bad bacteria that was causing illness, over time these bacteria became resistant to the effects of the medicine, making the impact of the drugs less effective or even completely ineffective. Not only did the antibiotics not work, but the bacteria grew stronger and could even make us sicker.

Research suggests that the early use of antibiotics is strongly associated with IBD development. In fact, when antibiotics are used in early childhood, there is an 84% greater chance of developing IBD than for those children who had not received antibiotics. [1] Also, the overall risk of developing IBD in association with antibiotics decreases as a child gets older. This suggests that antibiotics may indirectly affect a child's developing immune system by killing beneficial bacteria within the bowels.

Of course I am not suggesting that antibiotics should never be used to combat disease in kids. It only means that antibiotics need to be used judiciously, and the risks need to be weighed against their potential benefit.

---

1 Kronman MP, Zaoutis TE, Haynes K, Feng R, Coffin SE. Antibiotic exposure and IBD development among children: a population-based cohort study. *Pediatrics*. Oct 2012;130(4):e794–803.

What else affects what bacteria are in our intestines?

Food, drink, and anything else we put into our mouths affect our bacteria. We know this from a variety of examples. First, strong evidence exists that inflammatory bowel disease is affected by nutrient intake. A high total intake of dietary fats, polyunsaturated fatty acids, omega-6 fatty acids, and meats has been associated with an increased risk of Crohn's disease and ulcerative colitis; inversely, diets high in fiber and fruit are associated with a decrease in Crohn's disease. Examination of the fecal microbiome in people with different diets shows very distinct enterotypes of bacteria. What has also been proven is that changing an individual's diet can change the types of bacteria in his microbiome!

Second, industrialized countries like the United States have a much higher rate of inflammatory bowel disease. When people immigrate to the United States from less developed countries, they are very unlikely to have or ever develop IBD. All of that changes for their offspring, who have the same chance of developing IBD as people who have lived in the United States for generations. This is because, unlike their parents, first-generation children grow up eating the foods from the country in which they are born.

The exclusive enteral nutrition (EEN) formula-based diet

Nutritional therapy has been successfully used to treat Crohn's disease for over four decades. This therapy has not only been extremely effective, but it has similar remission rates as steroids, a potent immune modulator. Nutritional therapy usually means that the doctor prescribes exclusive enteral nutrition (EEN); patients drink only formula for 8 to 12 weeks until their symptoms subside.

This formula-based diet has wonderful promise, but it also can be difficult to implement for some children. Formulas are usually either drunk orally or put through a nasogastric tube. Not only are the remission rates equal to that of steroids, but the healing of the intestinal mucosa is much better with nutritional therapy. Unfortunately, this therapy is not used as much today as it should be because patients find it difficult to administer, and often a lack of support exists, both financially and physically, with formula-based therapy. With EEN, relapse is common once the nutritional therapy is discontinued unless appropriate immunosuppressive medication or the specific carbohydrate diet is begun.

The specific carbohydrate diet (SCD)

This brings us finally to the specific carbohydrate diet, or SCD. You can read about its history on pages 18–20. This diet was initially developed to treat celiac disease, which at that time, its cause was unknown. Only through insight and observation did healthcare providers and patients notice that when carbohydrates from grains were excluded from the diet (which also removed gluten), that symptoms improved.

Initially, healthcare providers did not realize that only grains containing gluten (such as wheat, barley, and rye) caused celiac. Consequently, the SCD allowed no grains at all and the diet's major carbohydrate came from ripe bananas. Celiac disease patients quickly improved on this diet, and Dr. Sidney Valentine Haas, a prominent academic pediatrician and a passionate proponent of SCD for celiac treatment, also used it for other intestinal tract disorders, including IBD. One of his patients was the daughter of a woman named Elaine Gottschall, who saw such dramatic clinical improvement in her daughter that she became a big supporter of the SCD. As knowledge and usage of the diet within the medical field waned, Gottschall, having seen the immense success of the diet on her own child, wrote a book, *Breaking the Vicious Cycle: Intestinal Health Through Diet*, and became the best-known advocate for the SCD.

Why did I become a strong advocate for the SCD?

In a few words: Because the diet WORKS! It reduces symptoms and in some cases even eradicates the need for medicine entirely. Where did I learn this? From observing my own patients and the success stories that come from them and their families. They talk, I listen, and then we all try to work out the best solution. I know individuals who have been on the SCD for decades and have done extremely well.

The SCD and nutrition are an important component in the health of IBD patients. The SCD is thought to work by modulating the harmful bacteria in the intestines. That said, more studies need to be done to prove this is true. So many unanswered questions still remain. For whom is it best suited? What are the most important components that make it work? Do different foods affect individuals differently? We can't—and shouldn't—stop using nutrition as a therapy, but we also have to continue to examine in detail the effects of nutrition on disease development and progression.

Although the SCD is a treatment method in which I have great confidence, like all treatment options, it may not be the right choice or effective for all. The benefits and downsides of dietary therapy need to be addressed early on. Therefore, if you remember only one thing from this entire book, it is that you, your child, your primary gastroenterologist, and your healthcare provider are a team. Knowing that is the most essential part in assuring that the medical care your child receives is the very best.

The Specific Carbohydrate Diet: What It Is and If It's Right for You

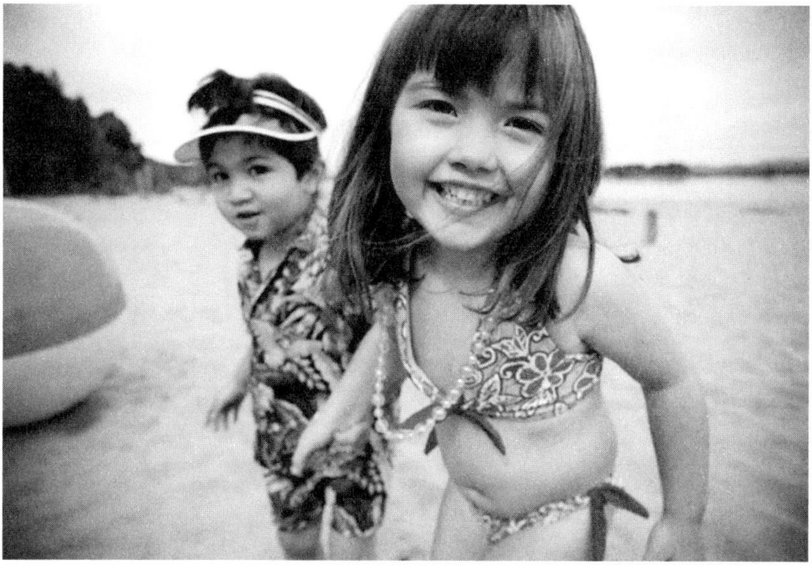

The Specific Carbohydrate Diet: Definition and History

What is the SCD?

The specific carbohydrate diet, or SCD, is a nutritionally balanced diet focused on removing grains, dairy except for yogurt fermented over 24 hours, and sugars except for honey. The diet focuses on natural, nutrient-rich foods, including vegetables, fruits, meats, and nuts. Individuals can still have breads and pastries, but the basis for such items is shifted from grain flours to nut flours, such as almond and coconut. Although its use and popularity began in treating celiac disease, it positive effects have now been shown in IBD as well.

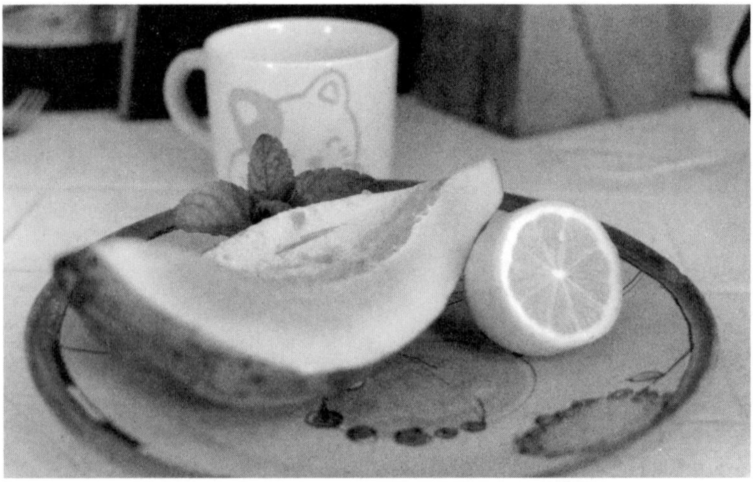

Early beginnings

The Specific Carbohydrate Diet (SCD) has an interesting history. Most people think it started with a report written over a hundred years ago by an English pediatrician named Dr. Samuel Gee. In 1888, Dr. Gee published an article wherein he described his patients with celiac disease. That's right, celiac disease—not inflammatory bowel disease. Dr. Gee would undoubtedly be surprised to see us reading about him now.

Aside from bringing celiac to the attention of the medical world, he made another important discovery: dietary treatment of celiac disease. "If the patient can be cured at all," wrote Dr. Gee, "it must be by means of diet ... the allowance of farinaceous food must be small."

Farinaceous foods? While the word "farinaceous" may be one we don't often use now, we know what it means: Farinaceous foods are ones that are heavily loaded with or solely consisting of particular starches such as those found in wheat, barley, rye, and spelt. Dr. Gee noted that when all grains or farinaceous foods were removed from the diets of celiac patients, they got better.

Dr. Gee had a keen mind. Through personal observation, he discovered the best way to treat celiac disease without even knowing why his method worked. He just knew it did. Now we know it's not all of the grains that are the culprits, but a specific protein found in *certain* ones—specifically gluten. Cheers to Dr. Gee for leading us in the right direction.

Dr. Gee's work influenced others as well. Dr. Luther Emmett Holt, a leading American pediatrician in the early 1900s, carried Dr. Gee's idea of restricting gluten to treat celiac disease even further, and his work went on to influence Dr. Sidney Valentine Haas in the 1920s. It is Dr. Haas to whom we give credit for taking everything that was then known and developing the guidelines for the specific carbohydrate diet or, as we call it, the SCD.

Dr. Haas, a pediatrician practicing in New York City, was also keenly observant. While he treated his young patients by restricting grains, he noted that many of them were able to tolerate fruits, certain vegetables, and even milk protein. In 1923, Dr. Haas proclaimed eight patients "cured" of celiac disease by way of a diet that excluded all carbohydrates except for bananas, specifically those with black spots on their skins. Excluded from the diet were breads, crackers, potatoes, and all cereals. Dr. Haas had still not identified gluten as the culprit, but his success with this diet occurred because of its exclusion. This specific carbohydrate diet, affectionately known as the Banana Diet, gained wide acceptance and popularity. Especially for people who liked bananas.

In 1951, Dr. Haas published his findings in a book called *Management of Celiac Disease*. In it, Dr. Haas further defined his own rendition of the SCD, and he did not restrict its use to patients with celiac disease but also prescribed it for patients with a variety of intestinal afflictions, including ulcerative colitis. One of these patients was Judy Gottschall, the daughter of Elaine Gottschall.

The dedication of a determined mother

Judy Gottschall had been diagnosed with ulcerative colitis at the age of eight. In an attempt to find a cure, Judy had been seen by a bevy of physicians, but all had found Judy's condition to be nonresponsive to medical management. Finally, as a last resort, it was suggested that the rapidly deteriorating Judy needed surgery—not a solution easily accepted by her mother, Elaine Gottschall.

Luckily, an answer was just around the corner. Judy and Mrs. Gottschall were referred to Dr. Sydney Haas, who put Judy on his specific carbohydrate diet. Slowly but steadily, her symptoms began to disappear. Elaine later became Dr. Haas's and the SCD's most passionate and energetic supporter.

In 1987, Mrs. Gottschall, who by this time had become well-known as a key proponent of the SCD, published *Food and the Gut Reaction*, which was republished in 1994 as *Breaking the Vicious Cycle*. At the time of its publication, no formalized study of the SCD on inflammatory bowel disease had been done; yet Mrs. Gottschall's book still has a strong following and continues to inspire people in the management of their IBD. It has also inspired numerous cookbooks that are geared specifically for the SCD.

SCD Food Philosophy

Importance of food

Hippocrates, the father of western medicine, is quoted as saying, "Let food be thy medicine and medicine be thy food." His insight, which is over 2,000 years old, still rings true today. In today's modern world, we often lose sight of the power of good nutrition and diet on our overall health and well-being. Food is medicine. We see this not only in diets like the SCD, which can resolve inflammation and help a person recover from debilitating symptoms, but also in all aspects of life and medicine. The healing effect of diet and nutrition is seen not only in inflammatory bowel disease but also in obesity, allergy, cardiovascular disease, seizure disorders, nonalcoholic steatohepatitis, chronic abdominal pain, and numerous other medical conditions.

But food also transcends medicine. Food is an experience. It tantalizes the senses: You can hear food as it cooks, see its rich colors, smell its magical aromas, and most importantly, taste it.

When starting the SCD, we sometimes are so wrapped up in the medicinal aspects of the diet that we lose sight of the actual food experience. The SCD introduces new and tasty foods, but it can sometimes be hard to see its full potential when you first start it. As you and your family move forward with the SCD, remember that a delicious world awaits that can heal you. Experiment and try new things … and dare I say—become a true foodie!

Eat whole foods only

A major part of good nutrition is to focus on whole foods. What does this mean? Eat foods that are either not processed or processed as little as possible. In our modern world, packaged foods are often manipulated to preserve their shelf life, improve their palatability and texture, and to enhance the short-term eating experience. When you eat whole foods, you avoid the potential for additives, which may have negative effects on your overall health. Whole foods offer other benefits as well, providing more complex micronutrients, essential dietary fiber, and naturally occurring protective substances, such as phytochemicals.

Eat organic

Organic foods are grown or raised without synthetic pesticides and chemical fertilizers. Organic meats, poultry, and eggs contain no antibiotics or growth hormones. Why eat organic? Unfortunately, no studies have been conducted proving or disproving the health effects and clinical benefits of organic foods; doing such studies are very difficult. A recent meta-analysis noted that "there have been no long-term studies of health outcomes of populations consuming predominantly organic versus conventionally produced food controlling for socioeconomic factors; such studies would be expensive to conduct."[2]

So, why organic? One clear benefit for avoiding meats from animals raised on antibiotics in their feed is the potential transmission of antibiotic-resistant organisms. The other is that we don't know the true safety and effects of synthetic pesticides, chemical fertilizers, antibiotics, and growth hormones in our food over the long term. But we do know that as these changes have occurred in our food production, we have seen an exponential growth in autoimmune disease cases in both children and adults.

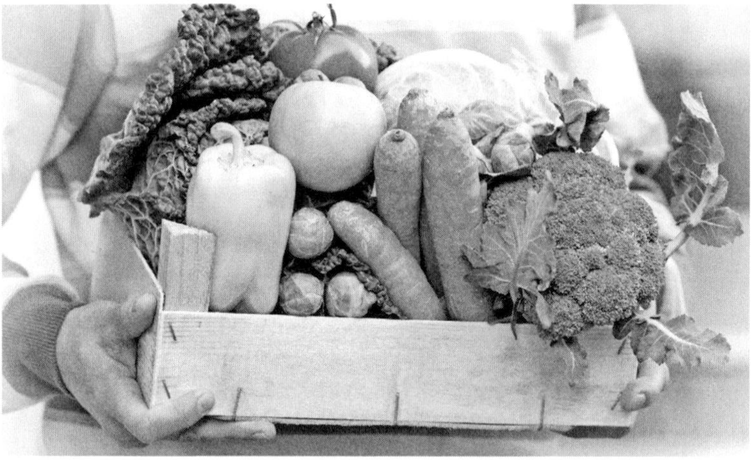

2 Smith-Spangler C, Brandeau ML, Hunter GE, Bavinger JC, Pearson M, Eschbach PJ, Sundaram V, Liu H, Schirmer P, Stave C, Olkin I, Bravata DM. Are organic foods safer or healthier than conventional alternatives?: a systematic review. *Ann Intern Med.* Sep 2012;157(5):348–366.

Experiment with ethnic cuisines

The SCD can appear very daunting in terms of restrictions. Fortunately, many cuisines exist throughout the world that do not use the restricted foods. You might, for instance, instead of focusing on SCD recipes, look at cookbooks and recipe websites that feature ethnic cuisines, such as southern Italian, Spanish, Indian, Middle Eastern, and southeastern Asian. You'll notice that these cuisines already have hundreds or thousands of recipes that fit the SCD with little or no alteration.

The recipes in this book are a starting point. As you use them, study various world cuisines and find the ones that fit the SCD and sound delicious to you and your family. Learn that cuisine's use of vegetables, meats, spices, herbs, and oils, as well as its cooking techniques. You'll notice that with some patience and an appreciation for whole foods, it is possible to create meals that are easy, delicious, and SCD-compatible.

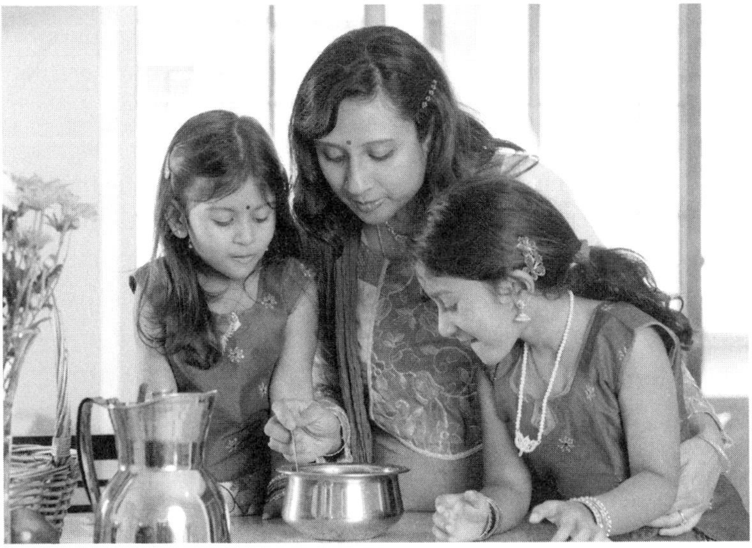

Is the SCD Right for You?

How to determine

The specific carbohydrate diet (SCD) oftentimes works with amazing end results for our patients. At Seattle Children's, we have seen great improvement and the disappearance of symptoms altogether for some. But others have experienced little or no improvement; it has not worked for everybody. While following the diet, some of my patients have been able to get off medications, while others continue to use the SCD in conjunction with their medical therapy. Many unanswered questions remain about how to integrate the SCD into one's healthcare plan. I am hoping that this book will be the first step in clarifying how to use the diet to ensure the best outcome for your child.

Do I recommend the SCD for everyone? The answer is a simple no. Whenever a decision on treatment is made for anyone, we always have to weigh the potential risks and benefits. What may be the right choice for one child is not always the right choice for another!

The SCD itself has no direct side effects. It can be a nutritionally balanced diet, but it still has many potential downsides that could occur. So it is important as a caregiver to be vigilant on how your child is doing. One of my major concerns is that individuals can get so engrossed in following the SCD that they lose sight of the symptoms that it is trying to treat. If the SCD doesn't work and disease activity goes unchecked, there can be serious negative consequences.

Determining if the SCD is right for your child is a personal decision that should always involve discussions with your healthcare provider. I use a number of criteria to help determine eligibility; this depends on the type of disease and the severity of the symptoms.

SCD and Crohn's disease

In the case of Crohn's disease, an individual with stricturing disease, severe perianal disease, or abscess or fistula formation should not rely on diet therapy alone as treatment. I don't recommend SCD as the sole therapy for individuals if they are experiencing severe symptoms of abdominal pain and diarrhea, or their pediatric Crohn's disease activity index (PCDAI) is greater than 65 (see page 185). In these situations, I often use concomitant medications to ensure that disease activity is completely under control.

Additionally, if children are failing to thrive or have stunted growth, especially if they are in their preteen or teen years (typically a time of rapid physiological growth), I feel that we should use a primary treatment in conjunction with the SCD, such as exclusive enteral nutrition (EEN).

When there are concerns among Crohn's patients that nutritional needs are not being met, EEN is a great option. This is a 100% formula-based nutrition, meaning that no other foods or drinks are allowed other than water. This has been shown to be just as effective as steroids to bring a person into remission, but the added benefits include better growth and weight gain. Using EEN also has much better intestinal mucosal healing rates than steroids. Although symptoms improve more quickly with steroids than with EEN, the actual mucosal healing is not as good as with EEN. This means that inflammation is still present, which puts individuals at a higher likelihood of relapse or flare. This much higher rate of mucosal healing means that EEN should be used for most people to treat their Crohn's. The difficulty with EEN is that it takes great commitment from the family and patient, but it works! The EEN is usually continued as the patient's sole food source for 8 to 12 weeks.

The PCDAI is a good thing for parents to know. It is an index that has been validated medically and statistically, and it defines an individual's disease activity. It gives parents and healthcare providers a way to objectively track disease and its severity (i.e., mild, moderate, or severe). This index is made up of clinical, physical, and laboratory criteria. The clinical criteria include abdominal pain, stools per day, and general well-being. The physical criteria include weight, height, abdominal exam, perirectal disease, and extraintestinal manifestations of disease, such as fever, oral ulcers, joint pain, and rash. The laboratory criteria consist of hematocrit, sedimentation rate, and albumin levels (see page 187 in "Laboratory Testing" in "How to Know If the SCD Is Working for You" for more information).

Because a parent or healthcare practitioner often does not have all this information on hand, it may be more helpful to follow the abbreviated PCDAI, which includes information on abdominal pain, well-being, weight, stool, abdominal exam, and extraintestinal manifestations but does not include the laboratory findings (see page 185 in "Which PCDAI Version Should You Be Using?" in "How to Know If the SCD Is Working for You" for more information).

If individuals have these exclusion criteria, it doesn't mean that they cannot do the SCD. It simply means that I would usually recommend the SCD in conjunction with standard medical therapy. Remember, it is always important to weigh the potential benefits and risks alike of any therapy in regard to how it will affect the disease and the severity of symptoms. The SCD can still be integrated into the treatment regimes that require standard medical therapy. Further down the treatment course, once the Crohn's disease has quieted, one may be able to get off of medical therapy and rely on diet alone. But this has to be decided on a case-by-case basis, and the risks and benefits need to be understood.

When the SCD may not work

Let's look at each of the different exclusionary criteria:

- **Poor growth.** Many children with Crohn's disease don't grow normally, and this affects both their height and weight. If the height and weight deficiency is significant and the child is in a period of fast growth, it's important that the child gets into remission in the most effective manner. This is because a growth deficiency in Crohn's can be permanent. For these children, nutritional therapy in the form of exclusive enteral nutrition (EEN) should be the number-one choice.

- **Abscess formation or fistulizing disease.** These issues need to be corrected using standard therapies. The reason for this is to avoid or lessen the need for surgical intervention, such as drainage and fistulectomy. Given the high likelihood of these symptoms progressing without standard treatment, the SCD by itself is not recommended.

- **Severe symptoms, or the PCDAI indicates severe disease.** It is important not to use the SCD in these cases. Why? Because it is critical that the patient gets better both physically and mentally in an effective, quick manner that has the highest likelihood of success. Does that mean your child can't do the SCD? Not at all, but I would bring an individual into remission with EEN or medication first. Long-term therapy with the SCD is still a viable option.

SCD and ulcerative colitis

What about ulcerative colitis? What would make me not use the SCD? The key is the severity of symptoms. If an individual needs hospitalization, a blood transfusion, or has a pediatric ulcerative colitis activity index

(PUCAI) greater than 60 (which indicates severe disease), I would not consider the SCD as a primary therapy.

The PUCAI is a score that is standardized and validated to assess disease activity in pediatric ulcerative colitis. It looks at clinical symptoms and can be a very helpful way to follow disease activity. It includes such factors as the number of stools per day, presence of blood in the stool, nighttime defecation patterns, abdominal pain, and well-being and activity level. The higher the number, the more severe the disease. And the more severe the disease, the more important it is to quickly get an individual into remission—and therefore treat with medications.

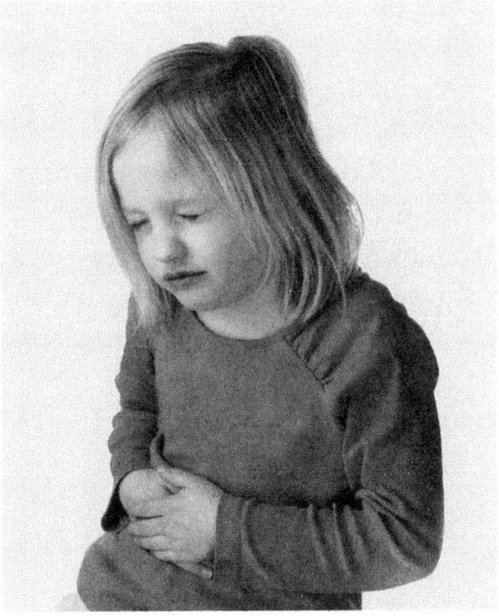

It takes sustained commitment

Outside of disease activity, there are other reasons to consider nondietary treatments. The first and foremost is that the SCD requires complete buy-in from all of the people involved—patients and family included. If compliance on the diet is not 100%, the patient is far less likely to enter remission. The second is time and energy; the family has to have enough of both to comply fully with the diet and integrate it into their life. It takes a lot of preparation to make sure that this diet works. This means buying the right foods and preparing them; we estimate that an extra half day every week is needed to ensure that the proper foods are obtained and made. The last major issue is time for improvement. The changes with SCD don't always come overnight; time and patience are an integral part of the healing process.

If you have read through this and you think you want to move forward with the SCD, make sure you have discussed the option with your gastroenterologist. It is important to build a team approach. Many gastroenterologists will be skeptical at first, because experience within the medical establishment with the SCD is lacking and not a lot of scientific data exists yet to prove to physicians that this diet works. But given time, there will be. We and others are working to show the benefits of this diet to others. Each patient who benefits from the diet helps transform the medical landscape, and this change will improve your gastroenterologist's perspective on the SCD.

The most important thing, whether your child is on the SCD or not, is that they are doing well. Their care has to be a team effort. Your gastroenterologist is a key part of that team. As people, whether we are parents, patients, or healthcare practitioners, we are all biased. We need to make sure our biases don't blind us from making appropriate healthcare choices. Making sure you properly discuss the benefits and risks of any therapy is key. We cannot reliably predict who will improve on this diet and who won't. Therefore, proper follow-up is crucial in ensuring that your child does well.

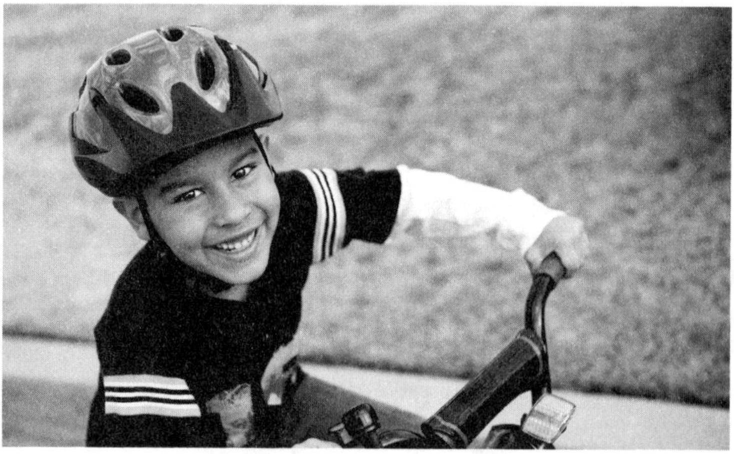

The Nutritional Adequacy of the SCD

How to determine

As a healthcare professional, I am always concerned about nutritional adequacy for a growing child. Nutritional adequacy is very important to ensure that children grow to their fullest potential (both literally and mentally), as well as to ensure that they have the energy to do all the things that they want. When I talk about nutritional adequacy, I'm speaking specifically about the components of the food that we eat. This includes the total number of calories; the amount of protein, carbohydrates, and fats in the diet; and vitamins and minerals.

When we first began using the SCD at Seattle Children's Hospital, we paid close attention to the food intake as well as the growth of the children whom we followed at their clinic visits. We noted when children appeared to grow well, gain weight, and thrive on the diet. We also examined certain foods that our patients were eating on the SCD and observed that, for the most part, individuals did take in enough calories, proteins, carbohydrates, and fats. Vitamin and mineral intakes were also largely sufficient for the majority of children, with the exception of vitamin D. Therefore, for children on the SCD at Seattle Children's, we recommend supplementing with vitamin D, based on the Institute of Medicine's dose recommendations.

Despite the fact that the patients we followed appeared to get enough overall calories, macronutrients, and micronutrients in their diet, we still make sure to discuss nutrition adequacy with families and children on the SCD. We have noticed that some individuals will focus on a few food types, such as fruits or certain SCD-approved foods, and they may eat a limited diet because they are not used to eating as many (or simply dislike) vegetables or meats. This is not limited to children on the SCD; many children in general are picky eaters and will limit their diets to only the food items they like.

This can be problematic if not addressed, because focusing on just a few SCD-approved foods can limit the amount of vital micronutrients ingested. Making this an open discussion is important to ensure that an individual is taking in enough macro- and micronutrients. This is also why following up with your healthcare provider as well as a registered dietitian who can analyze your child's nutrient intake for you is crucial. In addition, focusing on a few SCD-approved foods can sometimes lead to noninflammatory gastrointestinal complaints. This is especially true if your child consumes a lot of fruits and juices; the fructose within these foods, despite its being natural, can lead to bowel discomfort whether a person has IBD or not.

In essence, the SCD is nutritionally adequate, as long as you and your team are making sure your child is getting enough food and that food is varied.

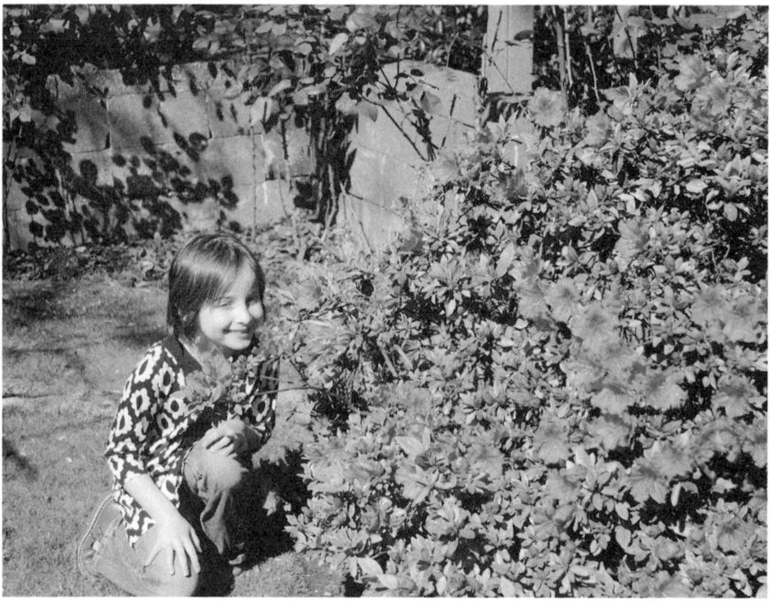

Getting on the SCD and Sticking with It

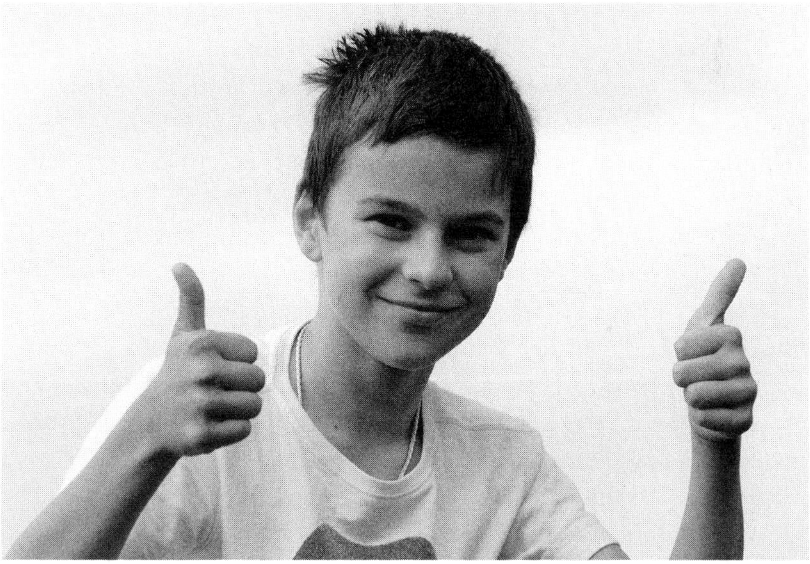

Family Stress

It can be hard

As a parent, a lot of responsibility and therefore a lot of stress falls upon our shoulders. We look at our children and want the best for them. We want them to grow up and experience life with joy and happiness.

Inasmuch, when loved ones develop chronic illness, whatever that diagnosis is, we to want to make it better and easier for them. This is especially true with inflammatory bowel disease and using dietary interventions to treat it. As parents, we often shoulder much of the burden in making sure our children do well. We check in with them on a regular basis; we remind them to take their medications or supplements; we help make sure that their friends, families, and healthcare providers understand what is going on with them; we try to make sure they are doing well now; and we continually think about and plan for their future needs.

With the SCD, another large responsibility is thrust upon you—that of making sure your child gets proper nutrition in and out of the house. This means learning a new way of cooking, shopping, organizing, and thinking. Initially, this can cause stress for your child as well as for you.

It is important to remember that all of these responsibilities and changes will not be easy at first. But stress is not necessarily a bad thing; in fact, in many instances, a little stress is quite a good thing. It brings a particular issue to the forefront and focuses us on getting things done.

But too much stress or stress that causes both mental and physical pain is a problem. Trying to get all the information you need in a very short time can be overwhelming. Stress that results in exhaustion, depression, or even anger needs to be avoided. This may sound obvious, but you need to be proactive in avoiding this stress. We especially see it in people without a supportive community, or when loved ones and family don't realize the amount of time and effort needed to make the SCD a possibility.

Another issue that can increase stress is when so much attention is being focused on just one child, while other children are being neglected.

While no magic bullet exists to solve all of these stressors, there are potential solutions.

It does get easier

First, realize that stress is absolutely normal. In our initial study, we asked individuals who began the diet what degree of stress they were carrying. Almost everyone was experiencing difficulty with starting the diet, but over time, their stress decreased dramatically. Time and experience gave everyone a better understanding of the diet, and what were initially challenges and hurdles eventually became routine and a daily part of life.

Take a break

Second, give yourself credit for all that you do and remember to give yourself a break. Although parenthood is a 24-hour, 7-day-a-week venture, finding some time for yourself is essential. Relax or exercise (I am a very big fan of exercise, as it has been shown to both decrease stress and improve overall health). Or do whatever you need to do to recharge.

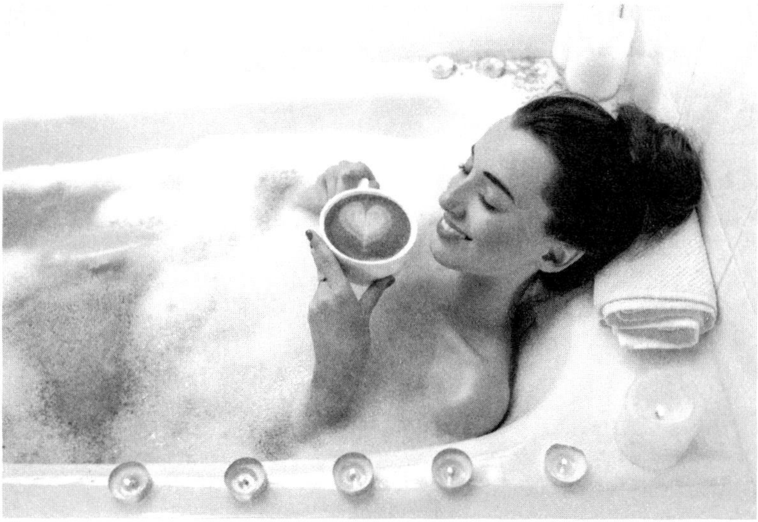

Join the IBD community

Surrounding yourself with a good support network and community is key to positively handling stress and staying successfully on the SCD. In my practice, I've had some families shop and cook for one another and share meal plans, thus dividing the labor involved in being on the SCD. Other SCD families get together on a regular basis for play dates and outings. It helps!

Many families of IBD patients at Seattle Children's have also joined the Facebook group "SCD families." This is a closed group (only parents of IBD kids are allowed to join). Not only do they share critical information on where to shop and what new recipes are available, but they also help one another balance life on the SCD, giving advice, support, and most importantly a sense of community. There are also many Internet forums for adults, which help form an important social structure for people on the SCD. (See page 80 for more information.)

Divide the work

Also, make sure that the SCD is a family affair. Dividing the tasks between family members can make the work much more manageable. Perhaps the father grocery shops, the mother cooks, and both parents along with their children do meal planning (or divvy up the jobs however it best works in your family). For single-parent families, it becomes a bit more difficult. Reaching out to friends and family is important. I have one family whose neighbors bake SCD muffins for them every week. Oftentimes the support structure already exists—a request for help just needs to be made.

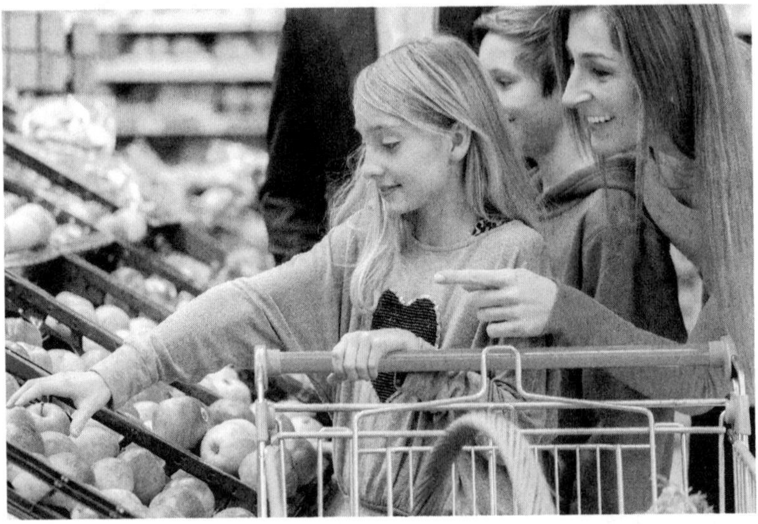

Involve—and empower—your child

Finally, make sure that your child is slowly but surely integrated into the knowledge and work of the SCD. What does that mean? Over time, you want your child to be able to do everything you are so that the diet is sustainable over the long term. To make this happen, they need to understand why they are on the diet, how it works, and the ins and outs of making the diet a success. As time goes on, have them help with the meal planning, shopping, cooking, and food preparation. As children become adults, they need to be prepared for this independence.

Children often want—and need—to feel empowered to make their own choices and have a say in their own destiny. It's almost always counterproductive for the parent to do everything for their children, and getting kids to take some responsibility for their own food choices makes it a lot easier on everyone.

Ending thoughts

So in short, stress is a normal part of starting the SCD. Remember to make sure you give yourself and your family kudos for making the SCD work, but just as important—give yourself a break for any bumps that may occur on the road.

A final stressor for the family is resistance on the part of the patient to being on the diet. This is especially true for some adolescents when the diet interferes with their social activities. It is absolutely important to hear your child and their concerns. If your child is completely against the diet and no workarounds will change their mind, listen to them. You can find a different treatment option while they are growing up. The SCD will be around for a very long time, and if it is not right for them now, they may find it right for themselves at a later time.

Important Food for Thought Regarding the SCD

1. Everyone in the family—parent and child—needs to be on board with the diet.

2. Changing one's lifestyle and diet is hard. Realizing that it is difficult for everyone to make the change and giving yourself time to understand the diet fully will ease some of the stress in starting it.

3. Everyone needs support. Find a sponsor! Find an SCD community! So many useful "tricks of the trade" can be learned from another person's or family's experience.

4. Make sure you follow up closely with your doctor.

5. Make sure you follow up closely with your dietician.

6. Many people won't understand what the SCD is or why you are doing this. This is okay; don't let it bother you. Ask your doctor to write a letter for your child stating that he is on a medically restrictive diet and should be allowed to bring in his own snacks and meals to the movies, restaurants, and the like (see page 75 for an example).

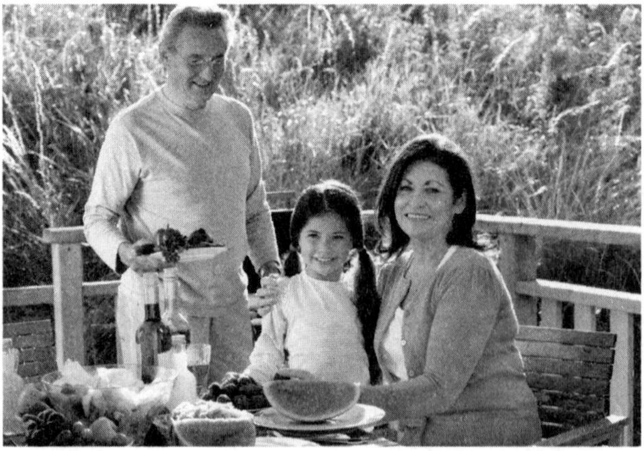

7. Educate other family members, such as grandparents. Their goal in life is to make your son or daughter happy, and sometimes they don't completely understand that no treats outside of the SCD really means no exceptions.

8. Continually praise your child for sticking to the SCD. It is hard on the parents who have to do the vast majority of food preparation, but staying on such a restricted diet is hard work, and your son or daughter deserves major recognition for this.

9. Continually praise yourself. It takes a lot of time to make this diet work for you and your family. Never forget to give yourself the kudos you deserve!

10. The most important thing is the health and happiness of your child, yourself, and your family. If the diet is too much of a hardship or causes too much stress or other unforeseen problems, talk about it with your healthcare provider. It is okay to go to medical therapy instead. There should never be guilt, shame, or blame if the diet does not work. Life is too short, and your child's overall health and well-being are the most important priorities, no matter which therapy is used.

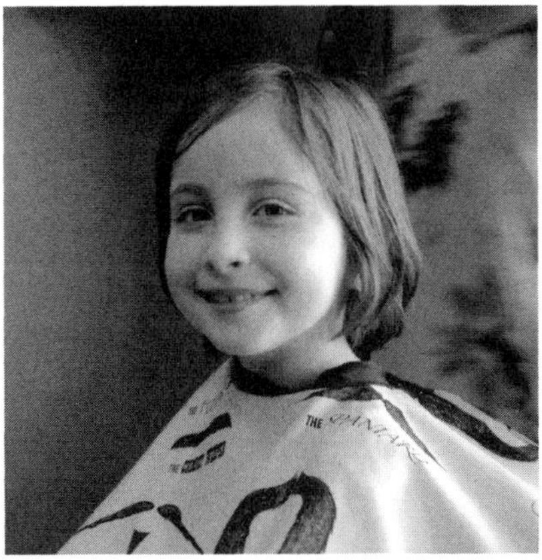

Our SCD Journey: Gil's and Tali's Story

In the winter of 2010, our 12-year-old son Gil was diagnosed with Crohn's disease. By then he had lost a lot of weight and was skin-on-bone thin, plus weak and exhausted from pain. Immediately after the diagnosis he started exclusive enteral nutrition (EEN), a medically supervised diet consisting solely of a nutritional formula. But staying on a liquids-only diet for 8 weeks, drinking Ensure and Pedialyte with no solid food whatsoever, was very hard on our child. His amazing self-discipline and compliance were fueled by the fear of having to endure more pain.

The EEN brought significant relief, but remaining on a liquid diet was no longer feasible. We needed a long-term plan, but we were hesitant about starting harsh medications at such a young age.

When we first read about it, the specific carbohydrate diet looked daunting and unsustainable, but some people on the Internet reported great results. We were skeptical and hopeful at the same time, and we decided to try it. Gil was a bit hungry during the first two days. Then he began to feel better and started enjoyed the soothing food: chicken soup, warm applesauce, well-cooked veggies with a bit of salt and butter. Gradually we added more SCD foods, and his diet became more varied, tasty, and nourishing. Within 2 months, his labs showed no inflammation markers. He gained weight and his energy came back.

I could finally stop the constant worrying that had kept me awake at night. We had a plan now, and it seemed to be working.

In the meantime, our kitchen had become command central. I was constantly cooking and baking, while my husband would pick up meat on his way home and help prepare it on weekends. The counter was always full of drying dishes, in addition to the dishwasher that was running twice a day. The kitchen work felt like that sorcerer's apprentice scene from the Disney *Fantasia* movie—it was never-ending and overwhelming.

Did my son's wellness mean a life sentence in the kitchen for me? At first it did. But necessity is the mother of innovation, and I learned ways to make things more efficient. With time and practice came a more sustainable kitchen load.

The SCD definitely forced some lifestyle changes upon us. We still spend a lot of time in the kitchen. We must plan, prepare, and pack food for everyday activities and before every outing. A daily lunch box for school, SCD snacks for afternoon sports, 3 days' worth of SCD foods for a road trip, and a week's worth of foods sent to summer camp—we do it all now with relative ease.

While the SCD seems restrictive, in actuality, it is the IBD that confines one's lifestyle. And the SCD allows our son to grow up free of IBD worries! He is now a junior in high school and has maintained the SCD for over 5 years. Like many teens his age, he is extremely busy with advanced classes, extracurricular activities, and preparations for college applications. The SCD keeps him well, allowing him to sustain this active and at times hectic lifestyle. He continues to enjoy good food and the freedom to be an active teen.

As we continue to learn more about the SCD, it is clear that the real challenges expand far beyond the steep learning curve of the diet's rules and demanding kitchen work. The emotional and social aspects of food are intricate, and they require awareness and preparedness when a child's wellness depends on compliance to a diet.

Some tips

Here are a few key points we wanted to share with fellow SCD parents:

If you see the obstacles, you took your eyes off the target

Be prepared for a possible moment when your teary-eyed child begs your permission for "just this once, I want pizza/ice cream/cupcakes like everybody else is having." On the SCD, every bite counts and there is no allowance for the wrong foods. As parents, it is our job to teach techniques for craving control: Never go hungry, self-distract by refocusing on other pleasant activities, or find an SCD food that is similar in texture or flavor to the forbidden food.

Remind yourself and your child that we all face challenges differentiating between what we want NOW and what we want MOST. For example, tell your child: "You want cake NOW, but if you let this craving pass, you will get what you really want MOST, which is a sense of control, freedom from the restrictions of IBD symptoms, and the energy to pursue your dreams."

Staying focused on this bigger target helps reduce the influence of a momentary craving.

Failing to plan is planning to fail

Always keep a variety of SCD treats in your freezer and in your pantry. Teach your child to never leave the house without taking SCD snacks in their bag, pocket, car . . . this is insurance against both social and emotional food temptation.

Let's say your child wants to meet friends for pizza and a movie at the mall. He can take a frozen SCD pizza out of the freezer, warm it, and eat it at home before leaving. This way he satisfies his "pizza fix" and he is not as hungry. He can then take with him an SCD muffin and a small plastic bag with nuts. When his friends order pizza, he can get a bottle of water and sit with everybody, sipping water, munching on his SCD muffin, and enjoying the conversation. Later at the movie, if friends order popcorn, he has the bag of nuts to munch on. With some preplanning, the social needs are met, and the diet is kept in full compliance.

"No, thank you!" is a full sentence

"This is SOOO good! I baked it myself! Try just one bite!" Whether it's a family member or a good friend, at some point a "food pusher" will be unavoidable. We must prepare our child ahead of time and practice at home on how to say "No, thank you!" politely but firmly. Our SCD child should not be apologetic about his diet, but rather feel very proud of it and the highly developed life skills that come with it. An ability to preplan from a young age, a well-developed sense of self-control, and some excellent eating habits—these are all well-earned gifts. Learning how to handle insistent food pushers is an extra bonus, as is practice in handling other challenging characters later on in life.

It's not about restrictions—it's about empowerment

The right state of mind can also support our SCD child through the challenges he might face with the diet. An inner dialogue that focuses on restrictions and deprivation is not helpful. The quality of our life depends on the quality of our thoughts. When talking and thinking about SCD, we should focus on the sense of empowerment it brings and the wellness it supports.

How to SCD Everyday

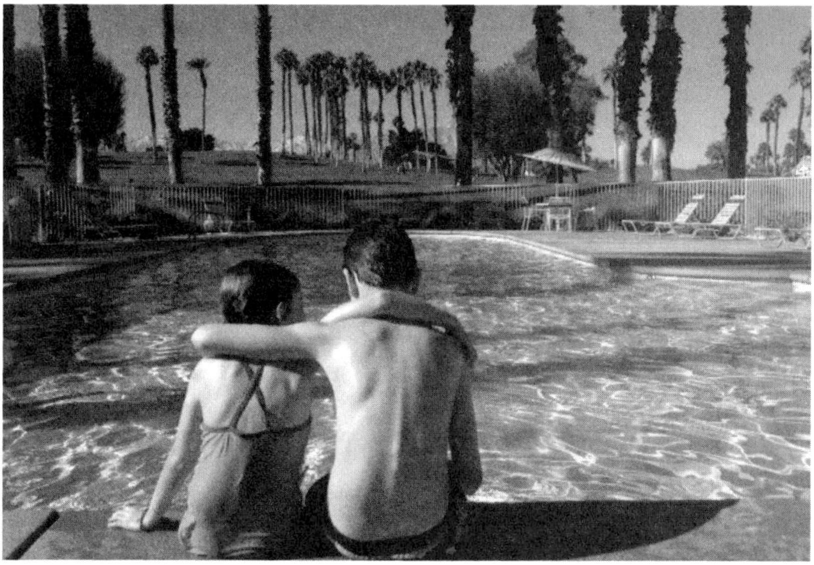

The SCD Stages

A step-by-step approach

The specific carbohydrate diet (SCD) is first and foremost a diet that removes all grains, milk products (except for highly fermented yogurt), and sugar from the diet. Many people have their own definition of what is legal and illegal on the SCD, and most of these food lists have been based upon people's personal and sometimes collective experiences.

At Seattle Children's Hospital, we divide the SCD into three main dietary stages, with each stage differing in terms of what can be eaten, its challenges, and how success is monitored. As with any intervention, it is important that during these three stages, an individual is closely monitored for overall well-being as well as nutritional status.

The three stages of the SCD:

1. Diet introduction and anti-inflammatory stage
2. Foundation and maintenance stage
3. Food reintroduction stage

Although different variations of the SCD have been around for over 100 years, the diet has not been studied extensively in medicine. The recommendations initially set up by Dr. Sidney Haas in the early 1900s were intended for individuals with celiac disease, and he later adapted the diet for inflammatory bowel disease using his clinical experience. Elaine Gottschall then adapted the diet and its recommendations based upon the experience of her daughter and others. Although this anecdotal experience may not completely answer all of the questions regarding the diet, it does show that this diet works for many.

For healthcare providers, patients, and their families, the difficult part is figuring out which steps of the SCD are the most important, as well as which steps are absolute and which ones can be modified for an individual. You will hear both a lot of different opinions as well as many different experiences with the SCD. Again, these experiences and opinions are important, as they make up the combined evidence that this diet works; but we must remember that each individual is different, and one person's experience may not mirror another's.

In my experience, I've seen many individuals do well, but also some who didn't. I've also seen patients who needed to be on a very strict diet without the ability to add new foods, while others were able to add a limited number of foods without difficulty. This is one reason that this book is being published—to help set guidelines for ourselves. And I have no doubt that as we study this diet further, our current recommendations will be refined.

When doing nutritional therapy, it is important to work with your healthcare professional as well as a dietitian to ensure that the SCD is working for you and that no complications are arising from the diet itself. To do this, we have set up a protocol for evaluating individuals on the SCD. This protocol really reminds us of what our goals are—good health and nutrition.

Stage 1: Diet introduction and anti-inflammatory stage

For individuals who are just beginning the diet and in the first stage (the anti-inflammatory stage), close follow-up is required on a regular basis. Prior to starting the SCD, both individuals and their families need to understand the diet, as well as prepare for the work that it entails. Once you begin the SCD, you should follow up with your healthcare provider in 1 to 2 weeks. During each visit, we recommend that patients review how they are doing and have a full physical, including a weight check. Laboratory studies such as complete blood count, sedimentation rate, C-reactive protein, and albumin should be checked as well (see pages 186–188 for more details).

During this time, your healthcare practitioner should check the PCDAI/PUCAI scores. What are these? They are validated scores for inflammatory bowel disease, meaning that you can then have an objective measure of how well your child is doing. This information can be helpful for healthcare providers, patients, and parents to help track how an individual is doing with a specific treatment.

For Crohn's disease, we follow the PCDAI, which is the pediatric Crohn's disease activity index. This score helps individuals determine if they are in remission or having mild, moderate, or severe disease activity. For score details, please refer to page 185 on PCDAI. For individuals with ulcerative colitis, we follow the pediatric ulcerative colitis activity index, or PUCAI (page 186). This is also a validated score for disease activity for children with ulcerative colitis.

These scores are very important. Although our memories may seem reliable, sometimes days, weeks, or months pass, and it becomes much harder to remember exactly what happened when. And if you follow these scores, you can have a much better understanding of how well things are going.

The goal of each checkup is good health and nutrition. Our expectation for these first visits with the healthcare professional is to ensure that individuals are maintaining their weight or at least have minimal weight loss. We also want to make sure that their symptoms are under control and that their laboratory studies are within an acceptable range. These follow-up visits can also be a good time for individuals to ask their healthcare providers and dietician about specifics in regard to the diet. We recommend scheduling clinic visits every 1 to 2 weeks to ensure that the child is doing well.

Stage 1 foods

At Seattle Children's, we practice a standard and practical approach to the addition of foods in the specific carbohydrate diet. When we initiate the SCD, we begin with Stage 1—diet introduction and the anti-inflammatory stage. We also return to this stage at the beginning of an IBD flare.

- **Homemade broth** is a staple of Stage 1. Chicken broth is the easiest to start experimenting with first, but turkey and beef-bone broth are also great choices, depending on your family's taste preferences. Broth can be either sipped by itself or mixed in a blender with cooked chicken and cooked vegetables to create a thicker soup or a savory smoothie. To date, no commercial SCD-legal chicken broth exists; please see page 136 for a recipe for homemade chicken broth.

- **Homemade applesauce** (using peeled, well-cooked apples) can be eaten cold or warm, with a bit of honey and cinnamon to taste. For extra calories, you can add coconut oil (*not* coconut butter, which is a food for a more advanced stage). See page 122 for a recipe.

- **Homemade SCD cultured yogurt and yogurt smoothies** made with very ripe bananas and cooked berries may also be included. If dairy products are a problem, this yogurt can also be made from homemade almond milk or coconut milk. See page 89 for a recipe.

- **Diluted fruit juice** (100% juice with no sweeteners or additives) is a beverage option. It can also be used to make a homemade gelatin dessert, using plain powdered gelatin.

- **Mock meat patties** can be made by combining one part cooked chicken with two parts of cooked green vegetables. See page 148 for a recipe.

- **Eggs** can be added with caution, after a day. An egg sensitivity might be present, especially at the beginning of the diet. But eggs, if tolerated, can be a versatile base ingredient for pancakes and other dishes:

  - Mashed banana and eggs for sweet pancakes.
  - Mashed vegetables and eggs for savory pancakes.
  - Mashed chicken and eggs for chicken pancakes.
  - Egg-drop soup is another good option, using homemade chicken broth and whipped eggs to create a savory and soothing breakfast.

It can be a lot of work to make these foods from scratch. But there are good reasons to! When a person is experiencing active disease symptoms, we want to make sure that there is no possibility that illegal foods or additives that may cause the diet to be less effective accidently get into the patient's meals. This vigilance gives the diet the best chance of success.

Stage 1 is often followed for just 1 to 2 days. During this period, a slight increase in abdominal discomfort often occurs; it is usually milder than the GI symptoms from an individual's IBD itself, and it is probably related to the "bad" bacteria dying off.

After a few days of being on Stage 1, you can move on to the regular SCD, gradually adding solid foods, including fresh fruits and vegetables, nut flours, lentils, and beans. Introduce only one new food at a time. A 2-day interval is a great (but not mandatory) guideline for introducing new foods. This will make it possible to determine whether each new food can be tolerated. Although the initial SCD did not break the diet into stages, many helpful guidelines exist online at resources such as www.pecanbread.com.

Stage 2: Foundation and maintenance stage

Once individuals start gaining weight and are seeing clinical improvements, we then decrease visits to every 2 to 4 weeks. We expect clinical remission within 2 to 3 months of dietary change. If we do not see this, we do not necessarily consider the diet a failure, but we will start thinking about why the diet is not working, as well as other therapeutic options available to us.

If an individual goes into remission, meaning that they are not only growing well and gaining weight but their symptoms have also abated, we then go to the diet foundation and maintenance stage, where we follow up with individuals on a 3- to 4-month time frame. We often monitor stool calprotectin levels to help ensure that no or minimal inflammation is present within the bowels.

If an individual is completely asymptomatic, with no evidence of inflammation on screening labs such as sedimentation rate and C-reactive proteins, but still has elevated stool calprotectin, we will often repeat endoscopy and colonoscopy procedures to evaluate true inflammation levels. This helps us appropriately focus our therapeutic interventions. Young children and individuals with IBD may have mildly elevated calprotectins that may not signify active disease. Therefore, it is important to interpret their calprotectin levels in the context of their age and how they are doing.

Stage 2 foods

In Stage 2, foods may be introduced in a stepwise fashion. Initially with food preparation, all vegetables and fruits should be peeled, seeded, and well-cooked. Within the fruit category, overripe bananas with brown spots as well as applesauce are allowed. Examples of vegetables to begin with include spinach, butternut squash, and acorn squash.

As individuals show signs of tolerating these additional foods, new items should be introduced every day or 2 days, such as green beans, peppers, mushrooms, avocados, tomatoes, peaches, pineapple, and plums. If no symptoms or flares occur, the diet can be expanded further (see the table below). Again, initially fruits and vegetables should be peeled, seeded, and well-cooked. Because new items should be introduced every day to 2 days, this initial step of Stage 2 can last 3 to 4 weeks. If the diet is moving forward well, raw peeled vegetables and fruits may be added. And if these are tolerated, then fresh, whole, unpeeled fruits and vegetables may be eaten.

- **Vegetables:** Asparagus, beets, bok choy, broccoli, Brussels sprouts, cabbages, carrots, cauliflower, celeriac, celery, Chinese cabbage, collards, cucumbers, eggplants, garlic, green beans, peppers, kale, leeks, lettuce, mushrooms, pumpkins, onions, parsley, spaghetti squash, Swiss chard, tomatoes, watercress, and winter squash.

- **Fruits:** Apples, blackberries, blueberries, cantaloupe, cherries, dates, elderberries, figs, gooseberries, grapefruits, kiwifruits, kumquats, lemons, limes, mangoes, oranges, papayas, passion fruits, peaches, pears, persimmons, grapes, strawberries, tangerines, and watermelon. Also dried fruit and raisins.

- **Meats:** Crisp-fried pork, SCD-legal bacon, meats battered with almond flour or deep-fried, and dried meats like jerky.

- **Nuts and seeds:** Split peas, lentils, lima beans, navy beans, black beans, and kidney beans; nut butters such as almond and pecan; nut milks such as almond, cashew, hazelnut, and macadamia nut; nut flours such as coconut, walnut, and macadamia nut; nut pieces and coconut flakes; and nut milks and homemade yogurts made from them, including coconut, blanched almond, and pecan.

Because this stage often goes well, close follow-up with the physician is not always required. But it is important that if any issues or concerns arise, you call your doctor so a plan can be made. And it can be definitely helpful to examine online resources, recipe sites, and cookbooks to get ideas that can add variety to your child's diet.

Stage 3: Food reintroduction

With the third stage of the diet comes so-called "illegal" food reintroduction. This is a very hotly debated step. Why? Because everybody has an opinion. With many of my patients, I am a purist and don't recommend adding any illegal foods. The difficulty with adding an illegal food is twofold: It may not only trigger a flare of the disease, but also some individuals, once they start adding new foods back in, cannot stop. I had a young lady who did extremely well on the SCD for over a year. She thrived so much that we decided to slowly add illegal foods per our protocol. She continued to do well both clinically and in her labs until she decided on her own to add Pop-Tarts. She soon flared.

This stage has no set time frame. Many individuals may not want to even consider limited reintroduction of a small number of illegal foods. The earliest I have ever reintroduced illegal foods was after 3 months on the diet; this was done for individual children who said that they could not maintain the strict SCD any longer. But other individuals have waited at least a year.

The most important aspect of this stage is to do things slowly and one step at a time. In addition, we very closely monitor symptoms and laboratory studies, as well as stool calprotectin levels to ensure that inflammation is not rebounding. Typically I will order a stool calprotectin test prior to initiating an illegal food, and then again 1 month after that food has been reintroduced. If the stool calprotectin significantly increases during that time, I will remove that food and recheck to ensure that these levels have normalized before restarting food introductions. As with all of these recommendations, adjusting for each individual's unique needs is important and often necessary.

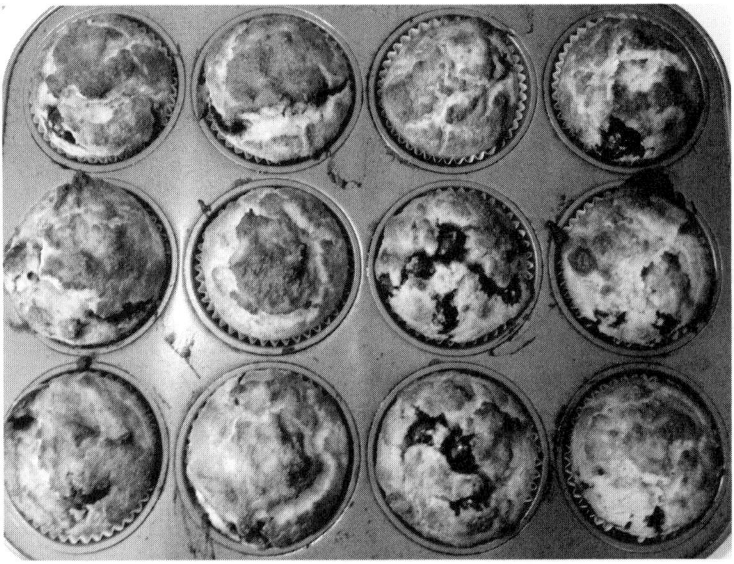

The SCD Process: A Graphic

Before starting the specific carbohydrate diet (SCD)

- Discuss with your primary gastroenterologist.
- Learn as much as you can.
- Become a part of an SCD community.
- Understand the food preparation and resources needed.

Begin the SCD

- Make sure you have a clinic appointment with a weight check and laboratory baseline values.
- Meet with your IBD clinic team, including your registered dietician.
- There can be some initial abdominal discomfort when starting the diet. This may be secondary to the body and microbiome adjusting to the SCD. This discomfort is usually distinct from IBD abdominal pain.

Week 2: Clinic follow-up

- Meet with your IBD clinic team, including your registered dietician.
- We expect a small amount of weight loss and mild improvement in clinical symptoms.
- If there are concerns about significant weight loss or significant clinical worsening, consider an alternative treatment plan.
- Repeat laboratory blood studies.

Week 4: Clinic follow-up

- Meet with your IBD clinic team, including your registered dietician.
- We expect continued clinical improvement, as well as improvement in laboratory parameters.
- Discuss with your healthcare team what seems to be working, as well as how to problem-solve any diet and nutrition issues.
- Be careful of the pitfall of eating the same things. Food diversity is important!
- If there are concerns for significant weight loss or significant clinical worsening, consider an alternative treatment plan.
- Repeat laboratory blood studies.

Week 8: Clinic follow-up

- Meet with your IBD clinic team, including your registered dietician.
- We expect continued clinical improvement, as well as improvement in laboratory paramenters.
- Discuss with your healthcare team what seems to be working, as well as how to problem-solve any diet and nutrition issues.
- If there are concerns for significant weight loss or significant clinical worsening, consider an alternative treatment plan.
- Repeat laboratory blood and stool calprotectin studies.

Every 3 months: Clinic follow-up

- It is important to continue to follow up with your GI providers. This is true even when you and your child are doing great.
- Continue to track laboratory tests, weights, and discuss how things are going with your healthcare team.

Meal Planning

It can be hard

Organized meal planning seems to be essential for families who are on the SCD, because it helps reduce a lot of the stress of going on the diet. With focused meal planning, people develop an understanding of what is needed in terms of groceries, which leads to less redundancy of foods. It also helps promote a greater variety of meals, as parents can see what has been eaten most recently. And it gives children an opportunity to have more of a say in what they are eating, which can help foster their SCD independence.

Another positive aspect of meal planning is that it allows individuals to plan for busy days. Meals can be prepared ahead of time (on the weekends, for instance), and frozen or stored in advance. Advance food preparation, like always having veggies chopped up in baggies or soup frozen as ice cubes, can save valuable time and frustration in harried moments. This can decrease the stress of having to make SCD-appropriate meals or snacks in a pinch or when time is tight.

There are many ways to meal plan, and lots of great online resources are available to help with that. What has worked well for many of the families at Seattle Children's is to make a weekly or biweekly meal plan. This enables IBD individuals and their parents to prepare not only a variety of meals throughout the week, but also to make sure that enough snacks and goodies are available for nibbling. In addition, families can divide the work, with some individuals doing the shopping while others prepare the food.

Effective meal planning needn't be hard, and you can do it lots of different ways. First, decide what meals and foods you want to serve over the upcoming week or two weeks. This means thinking about the dishes and recipes that you and your family like. It can be helpful to have a number of cookbooks or recipe websites available to help inspire you with ideas. Write out the names of these dishes. Then, on another piece of paper, write the shopping list based on these dishes. It may also be useful to record these on a calendar. As time goes on, the family can see and rate what dishes they liked (or didn't), and which ones should be made again.

It's important when doing meal planning to realize that people eat more than just breakfast, lunch, and dinner, and that snacks are an integral part of meals during the day. Write these out as well. You and your family should grade them too.

Remember that in meal planning, variety is the spice of life. A whole array of foods that are SCD-approved is awaiting you. These foods should be explored! As time goes on, you'll accumulate a large number of recipes, and meal planning will be easier, even second nature.

Sample meal plans by SCD stage

How restrictive you have to be when starting the diet will depend on how well your child feels. Here are three sample meal plans for Stage 1. It is best not to insist on formal mealtimes in the first days. Instead, encourage your child to eat and drink small portions throughout the day, as often as is comfortable.

Sample SCD Stage 1 meal plan for 3 days

Stage 1 — Sample Meal Plan for Day 1

Day 1 needs to be egg- and dairy-free.

Mix and match multiple small servings from the list below and offer through the day:

- Homemade chicken broth, turkey broth, or beef bone broth (alternate if you aim for variety).
- Homemade apple or pear sauce.
- Diluted SCD-legal apple or grape juice (half juice, half water).
- Homemade gelatin made from organic, powdered gelatin and diluted grape or apple juice.
- Chicken soup (including chicken pieces and carrots). Chew the food well.
- Chicken-vegetable patties (finely ground cooked chicken and cooked vegetables).
- Chicken-vegetable puree (finely ground cooked chicken and carrots in a small amount of homemade chicken broth).
- Ripe, brown-speckled banana (can be cooked with a dab of butter or coconut oil to a creamy consistency).

Stage 1 — Sample Meal Plan for Day 2

Day 2 can include eggs.

Breakfast

- Homemade broth with egg-drop swirls
- Chicken-veggie patties
- Diluted juice or diluted gelatin

Snack

- Homemade applesauce
- Banana-egg pancake

Lunch

- Chicken-veggie patties
- Zucchini strips (peeled and deseeded, cooked or baked with a dab of butter or coconut oil)

Snack

- Diluted gelatin

Dinner

- Chicken soup (including the cooked chicken and carrots)
- Homemade applesauce

Menus courtesy of Tali Guday, of Gut Harmony.

Stage 1 — Sample Meal Plan for Day 3

Day 3 can include eggs and yogurt.

Breakfast

- Veggie-egg pancake (made from finely ground cooked veggies mixed with egg)
- Homemade applesauce

Snack

- ¼ cup homemade SCD yogurt, flavored with a drop of honey and topped with a two spoons of strained berry puree. (Cook and strain a whole bag of frozen berries through a fine-mesh strainer; discard the seeds and peel. Keep the smooth puree in a refrigerated jar. Gradually increase the amounts of yogurt in the coming days if it is well tolerated.)

Lunch

- Chicken soup (including chicken pieces, cooked carrots, and peeled, deseeded zucchini)
- Homemade gelatin dessert made from organic, powdered gelatin and diluted juice

---

Snack

- Banana pancakes
- Diluted mint tea or juice

Dinner

- Chicken-veggie patties
- Homemade gelatin dessert made from organic, powdered gelatin and diluted juice

---

Sample SCD Stage 2 meal plan for 1 day

Stage 2 — Sample Meal Plan for 1 Day
Breakfast • Poached eggs • SCD-legal bacon • Grape juice (diluted half-in-half with water)
Snack • Fresh blueberries • Almond milk
Lunch • Tomato soup • SCD-legal crackers • Spinach and egg flan • Fresh peaches
Snack • Vegetable nuggets with hazelnut dip • Cranberry juice (diluted half-in-half with water)
Dinner • Tomato soup • Pecan-crusted orange roughy • Butternut squash • Caramel-pear upside-down cake

Sample SCD Stage 3 meal plan for 1 day

Stage 3 — Sample Meal Plan for 1 Day

Breakfast

- Mushroom-and-leek scrambled eggs
- Sliced mango
- Orange juice

Snack

- Fresh cantaloupe
- Almond milk

Lunch

- Caesar salad
- Sloppy joes with SCD-legal buns
- Zucchini al limon

Snack

- Savory muffins
- Coconut milk

Dinner

- Spinach-artichoke dip with mushrooms, onions, and roasted red peppers
- Braised beef with fennel
- Cauliflower couscous
- Almond cake

Sample SCD Stage 3 meal plan by week

Day 1

Breakfast

- Braised chicken omelet
- SCD yogurt with fresh mango

Lunch

- Seared and sliced chicken strips
- Roasted zucchini and carrots
- Butter-and-almond-flour rolls

Dinner

- Spaghetti squash "vermicelli" with beef meatballs and marinara sauce on the side
- Honey-and-coconut-flour macaroon cookies

Snacks

- Pear sauce with lentil crackers
- Vegetable nuggets with hazelnut dip

Day 2

Breakfast

- Almond- and coconut-flour banana pancakes with honey butter
- Hand-ground pork sausage with onion and fennel seed

Lunch

- Red lentil "tortillas"
- Caesar salad

Dinner

- Braised chicken thigh and legs with salt and pepper
- Mashed white beans and cauliflower with butter and chicken jus
- Asparagus with lemon and parsley
- Date-and-apricot cake with coconut-and-honey icing

Snacks

- Black-bean tortilla chips with salsa and white-bean hummus
- Banana snack with peanut butter, honey, and almonds

Day 3

Breakfast

- Ham and cheese omelet
- Blueberry almond-flour muffins

Lunch

- Baked chicken strips
- SCD-legal hot dogs with steamed-lentil buns

Dinner

- Stir-fried shrimp with garlic, ginger, zucchini, squash, carrot, and sesame oil
- Sesame- and ginger-roasted broccoli

Snacks

- Cheesy cauliflower-crust flatbreads
- Old-fashioned tuna salad

Day 4

Breakfast

- Banana-bread-and-brown-butter french toast with honey butter

Lunch

- Seared and roasted prime rib with beef jus, black lentils, and almond-butter rolls
- Sautéed summer squash with herbs

Dinner

- Ground turkey taco meat with yellow-lentil tortilla chips
- Cuban spiced black beans
- Steamed broccoli and carrots with lemon olive oil
- Pear-sauce cookie with dried cranberries

Snacks

- Applesauce with lentil crackers
- Raw vegetables with lemon aioli

Day 5

Breakfast

- Scrambled eggs with butter and cheese
- Almond-flour toast made with whipped egg whites

Lunch

- Lentil-flour cheese dumplings with tomato sauce
- Grilled vegetable skewers with onion, mushroom, pepper, and zucchini

Dinner

- Beef burgers with lentil- and almond-flour buns
- White bean salad with carrot, onion, olive, peas, celery, and homemade mayonnaise (egg and olive oil)
- Lemon and vanilla cake with Swiss meringue frosting

Snacks

- Black bean chips with creamy tomato dip
- Fresh strawberries with SCD coconut-milk yogurt

Day 6

- Hand-ground pork sausage
- Almond- and coconut-flour banana pancakes with honey butter

Lunch

- Peppery vegetable soup
- Halibut with mango salsa

Dinner

- Cauliflower crust pizzas with cheese and sausage
- Sliced almond flour mini-biscuits for meats and cheeses
- Black bean brownies

Snacks

- Steamed lentil dumplings with honeyed SCD yogurt
- Homemade applesauce

Day 7

Breakfast

- Mediterranean melon with honey yogurt
- Bacon bites with cheese

Lunch

- Baked spaghetti squash with two cheeses
- Thai carrot soup

Dinner

- Sweet and sour pork
- Oven-baked crispy kale
- Apple upside-down cake

Snacks

- Spinach and egg flan
- Radishes with salt and butter

Table of SCD-Legal and Illegal Foods

What follows is a basic chart of SCD-legal and illegal foods, adapted from www.pecanbread.com. For a very comprehensive, searchable list of specific foods and ingredients, see the Breaking the Vicious Cycle website at www.breakingtheviciouscycle.info/legal/listing.

Allowed (Legal) Foods	Not-Allowed (Illegal) Foods
FRUIT	
All fresh, unprocessed fruit, based on the SCD stages. Organic is preferred. Applesauce should be homemade (recipe on page 122); do not use commercial applesauce.	Canned or dried fruit processed with additional sugar and additives.
VEGETABLES	
The vast majority of nonstarchy, unprocessed vegetables, including mushrooms. Organic is preferred. See the Breaking the Cycle website's Legal/Illegal List for complete details on individual vegetables.	Starchy vegetables, including white potatoes, sweet potatoes, rutabagas, parsnips, and yams. Any vegetable processed with additional sugar and additives. No canned or processed tomatoes or tomato products. See the Breaking the Cycle website's Legal/Illegal List for complete details on individual vegetables.

Allowed (Legal) Foods	Not-Allowed (Illegal) Foods
MEAT	
All fresh or frozen meats without SCD-illegal ingredients. Check the labels carefully for additives in solutions. Organic is preferred. Beef, lamb, pork, goat, buffalo, venison, wild game, rabbit, veal, liver, kidney, oxtail, tongue, and tripe are allowed.	All processed meats and meat products, such as cold cuts, hot dogs, bacon, sausages, dried beef, smoked meats, and Spam. Any meat processed with additional sugar and additives, including solutions.
POULTRY	
All fresh or frozen poultry without SCD-illegal ingredients. Check the labels carefully for additives in solutions. Organic is preferred. Chicken, turkey, quail, duck, and goose are allowed.	All processed and breaded products, such as chicken nuggets and canned products. Any poultry processed with additional sugar and additives, including solutions.
FISH AND SHELLFISH	
All fresh and frozen fish and shellfish, as long as it is unprocessed and unbreaded without additives. Canned tuna packed in water or in its own juices is legal. Sashimi is legal, but not sushi rice.	Any seafood processed with additional sugar and additives, including solutions.

Allowed (Legal) Foods	Not-Allowed (Illegal) Foods
EGGS	
All types of eggs are allowed, preferably organic and free-range.	
MILK, CREAM, AND BUTTER	
Plant-based milks, such as almond and coconut. Ghee, pastured-cow or "grass-fed" butter.	Milk from animals is not allowed. No kefir or margarine. No milk- and cream-based products (although it is okay to use these to make the homemade SCD yogurt).
CHEESE	
Hard cheeses aged over 90 days (Cheddar, etc.). No soft cheeses except dry curd cottage cheese (DCCC).	No soft cheeses, including ricotta, goat cheese, feta, cream cheese, mozzarella, and all other soft cheeses other than dry curd cottage cheese (DCCC).
YOGURT	
Homemade yogurt only. Use SCD guidelines for making yogurt from cow and goat milks, coconut milk, and nut milks. See pages 87–90 in "Making SCD Yogurt" in "Preparing SCD Food."	No commercial yogurts.

Allowed (Legal) Foods	Not-Allowed (Illegal) Foods
GRAINS, BREADS, AND CEREALS	
	No grains of any kind, such as wheat, rice, corn, quinoa, millet, amaranth, buckwheat, amaranth, teff, barley, spelt, rye, oats, and triticale. No products derived from these grains (such as pasta, cereals, crackers, breads, other baked goods, and many vegetarian meat substitutes).
SEEDS	
Generally allowed based on the SCD stages, including pumpkin seeds, with some exceptions.	Flax, chia, and hemp seeds are not allowed.
NUTS	
All nuts, including almonds, walnuts, pecans, cashews, hazelnuts, macadamias, peanuts, etc. Coconuts and coconut milk are allowed. All-natural nut butters may be better tolerated during the initial stages.	None with an SCD-illegal starch coating or that possibly has illegal ingredients used in the roasting process (as is the case with most commercial mixed nuts).

Allowed (Legal) Foods	Not-Allowed (Illegal) Foods
BEANS AND LEGUMES	
Only dried navy beans, lima beans, black beans, cranberry beans, green (string) beans, lentils, split peas, and regular peas cooked per SCD rules.	No garbanzo, kidney beans, and pinto beans. No canned beans of any kind. No soy in all forms.
HERBS AND SPICES	
All individual herbs and spices are legal. Onion powder and garlic powder are allowed as long as they are additive-free (such as anti-caking agents).	Avoid spice mixtures; buy spices separately.
CONDIMENTS, DRESSINGS, AND VINEGARS	
Homemade condiments and dressings without SCD-illegal foods are legal. Recipes are available online and in specialized cookbooks (see the Resources section on page 80). Most vinegars are legal except balsamic vinegar (except homemade; some recipes exist online).	No commercial condiments or dressings. No balsamic vinegar, except homemade.

Allowed (Legal) Foods	Not-Allowed (Illegal) Foods
SWEETENERS	
Honey is allowed. With artificial sweeteners, only Sweet'N Low is permitted (saccharine-based).	None except honey. No agave or stevia. No cane sugar (including raw, brown, white, or rapadura) or molasses. No date, coconut, or other palm sugar. No fructose, glucose, dextrose, sucrose, and isoglucose. No syrups such as maple or corn syrup. No artificial sweeteners except Sweet'N Low (saccharine is allowed but it is possibly not healthy).
FATS AND OILS	
Ghee, pastured-cow or "grass-fed" butter. Coconut oil, sunflower oil, olive oil, and all nut oils. All seed oils (sesame, peanut, canola, flaxseed, corn, and grapeseed).	No vegan butter products or soybean oil.

Allowed (Legal) Foods	Not-Allowed (Illegal) Foods
FERMENTED FOODS	
Sauerkraut, kimchi, pickles, and other fermented foods are allowed as long as they are made without SCD-illegal foods or added sugar.	Do not use commercial products with additives, preservatives, sugar, and other SCD-illegal foods.
BEVERAGES	
Freshly squeezed fruit and vegetable juices are allowed. Sparkling water is allowed. Most teas and coffee are allowed. See the Breaking the Cycle website's Legal/Illegal List for more details. Wine and whiskey are legal, while brandy and sherry are not. See the Breaking the Cycle website's Legal/Illegal List for more details on individual alcoholic beverages.	No fruit or vegetable juice made from concentrate or with additives. No soda of any kind.
CANDY AND CHEWING GUM	
	None are allowed, including chocolate, carob, licorice, and marshmallows. The one exception is that some families have done well with Wellbee's Pure Honey Candy (www.wellbees.com/pure-honey-candy-3318.html).

Allowed (Legal) Foods	Not-Allowed (Illegal) Foods
BINDERS, THICKENERS, ADDITIVES, AND OTHER	
Unflavored gelatin, baking soda (but not powder), and cellulose (in supplements only) are allowed.	No preservatives of any kind. Agar, carrageenan guar gum, potato flour, rice flour, and sorghum flour are not permitted. No whey powder, FOS (fructooligosaccharides), seaweed or seaweed products, algae (like spirulina and chlorella), arrowroot, baker's yeast, baking powder, cellulose gum, cornstarch, cream of tartar, dextrose, hydrolyzed protein, mastic gum, natural flavors, pectin, Postum, sago starch, tapioca, and xanthan gum.

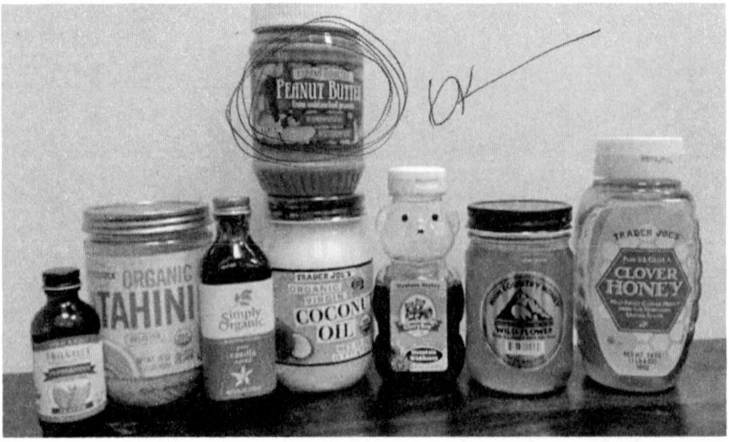

Making SCD Work Outside the Home

SCD at school

504 Plan

A 504 Plan is worthwhile whether your child is on the SCD or not. A 504 Plan refers to Section 504 of the Rehabilitation Act and the Americans with Disabilities Act, which specifies that no one with a disability can be excluded from participating in federally funded programs or activities, including elementary, secondary, or postsecondary schooling. This includes illnesses or injuries as well as chronic conditions like asthma, allergies, and IBD. Depending upon the support you have from school officials, staying on the SCD during school hours can be challenging, and having a 504 Plan in place can help your child comply.

Here are two common accommodations that will help support your student:

- **"Late arrival"** allows your child to skip first period, which, in middle and high school, begins very early in the morning. It allows more time to prepare and eat a proper breakfast at home before going to school. Eating breakfast and maintaining a consistent energy level is key to preventing "cheating on the diet" at school. But be aware of the possible drawbacks of this option:

    - With late arrival, the school bus is not available, which often results in the parent needing to drive the child to school.

    - To insure academic needs are met in middle and high school, some families choose to supplement the curriculum using online classes. For example, one high schooler on the SCD took five classes per semester at the high school and one class per semester online, via Brigham Young University.

- **"Permission to access, carry, and eat snacks in class."** Since backpacks are typically stored in hallway lockers, it is important to ensure access to food whenever the child feels they need it. This helps when an impromptu pizza party is held in class, or when a box of cookies is shared in the classroom (which happens a lot in high school). With proper permission in place, your child can go get an SCD snack from his or her backpack when these situations arise.

SCD and athletics

Sports is an important part of life for many children. Being on the SCD should not stop individuals from participating and excelling in whatever athletic endeavors they choose. Most of the time, having adequate snacks and hydration available is enough to maintain a child's physical activity. But for children with IBD, having a sufficient supply of high-energy foods and balanced electrolyte solutions can be especially important. Fortunately, nature gives us many of these foods—bananas and oranges, for instance, are great sources of calories and nutrients.

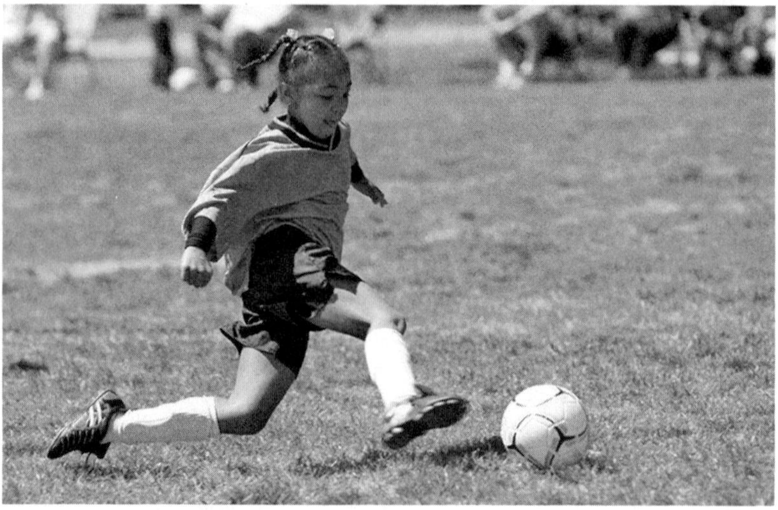

Extra food and emergency snacks

Make sure to pack extra food and snacks daily, and include SCD muffins, cookies, crackers, or other treats as insurance against non-SCD temptations.

In addition to SCD food in the lunch box, it is a good idea to have an emergency snack available in a pocket of your child's backpack. This must be a nonperishable item like a fruit leather bar, a bag of seeds and nuts, or some SCD beef jerky. It is handy for days when unexpected delays may raise a need for food before getting home (e.g., staying late at school to coordinate a last-minute class project, or if the school bus is delayed). An extra SCD snack will keep energy up and temptation at bay.

Important! Be sure to check that the emergency snack is in place on a daily basis (your child might forget to tell you that it has been eaten). Replace the snack often. This also ensures that it didn't spoil or that it didn't turn into an unappetizing, squished mush at the bottom of the backpack.

Packing and container strategies

Keep a collection of different sizes and shapes of lunch boxes, thermos cups, and water bottles. These are not just for school, but also for sports, evening outings, parties, etc. Having a variety on hand ensures that packing food in a hurry is easy and not stressful, and if a lunch box is forgotten at school, there is another one available for the next day. In addition, have several different types of lunch bags and carriers available, besides the individual containers that go inside them. These carriers should be in various sizes for any sort of outing, such as small and discreet for a movie theater, or larger for a picnic outing or school lunch.

SCD and eating out

Food is not only important to ensure proper growth and development, but it is a profoundly social activity. As children and adults, we like to sit around the table "and chew the fat," so to speak. Being with friends and family during meals is important, but being on the SCD and eating out can be difficult. Different people address this issue in different ways. It is important to remember that everyone's levels of sensitivity are different, and therefore dining out involves caution and some advance planning.

Bringing your own food ensures that what you are eating is truly SCD safe. As mentioned before, you can ask your healthcare provider for a letter to ensure that whatever restaurant or other venue you visit won't give you a hard time.

Some restaurants, especially nicer establishments that focus on customer satisfaction or healthful dishes, may be able to accommodate the SCD fairly easily. It is important to properly communicate with them (ahead of time if necessary) to make sure that eating out will be feasible. Salads, vegetables, fish, and other foods are doable! But avoid complex dishes and sauces in which unknown ingredients may lurk.

If you live in an area with others who are on the SCD, it might be worthwhile patronizing a few local restaurants who know about and can accommodate the diet. Just as there were almost no restaurants 15 years ago that provided gluten-free foods and now a plethora of them exist, so it can be with the SCD. Raising awareness by politely asking restaurants to create SCD-safe dishes is a way each of us can help change society and improve our dining climate.

Travel

The basics

- **Always carry an official letter (see page 75) from your doctor stating your need to be on a medical diet and to carry your own food.** Make a few copies—it may be useful at places such as restaurants and movie theaters.

- **If carrying yogurt will be a hassle, plan ahead and order SCD-legal probiotics to use instead of yogurt.**

- **Take any necessary medication or supplements in their original containers.**

- **Always take more food than you think you may need.** Carry water bottles and nonperishable snacks in your pocket or personal backpack *in addition* to the food in the coolers. Travel days make people more hungry than on a routine day. Extra food is also an insurance in case of unexpected delays and other mishaps.

Air travel

- **Plan ahead and prepare food suitable for carrying and consuming before, during, and after flights.**

- **Check ahead with the airline regarding current restrictions on carry-on bags and content,** to ensure that liquid food items will not be confiscated. Make sure you have your doctor's letter handy as well, to show security officials if necessary. Plan to take food that is allowed.

- **Also, don't forget to check the security and customs regulations in your country of destination in advance,** again to ensure that food items will not be confiscated upon arrival. Different countries have different regulations.

Packing list for an SCD road trip

- An SCD letter from your doctor (see the example on page 75): "*This individual must maintain a therapeutic diet and must be permitted to carry his own safe food.*"

- **Snacks**
  - Water bottles
  - SCD-legal fruit juice
  - Hard cheese cubes
  - Dehydrated beef jerky
  - Fruit leather
  - Legal LaraBars
  - Dried fruit and nuts
  - Fresh fruit and cut veggies
  - Hard-boiled eggs
  - SCD cookies and crackers in airtight containers

- **Frozen SCD main dishes**
  - Veggies
  - Soups and stews
  - Meat patties

- **Breakfast**
  - Frozen pancakes (portioned daily servings in zipper-lock storage bags) with cooked fruits and honey
  - Eggs
  - Sausage
  - Tea bags

- **Other items**
  - Pickles
  - Canned fish and chicken
  - Salt, pepper, and other seasonings

- **For the hotel**
  - Probiotics, *S. boulardii*, and other key supplements (keep cool or refrigerated)
  - An electric hotplate with a pot to heat liquids and a skillet for eggs, or an electric frying pan to heat liquids and cook or reheat foods
  - A Pyrex or ovenproof glass dish to warm frozen SCD meals (small enough to fit in a tiny hotel microwave oven)
  - Mugs
  - Spoons and forks
  - A small sharp knife
  - Picnic plates
  - Aluminum foil or parchment paper
  - Small zipper-lock storage bags
  - Large zipper-lock storage bags (to replenish ice cubes in car coolers)
  - Paper towels
  - Sponge and dish soap

- **In the car**
  - Hand sanitizers
  - Several coolers with ice packs (to keep these cool, every morning place new zipper-lock storage bags full of ice from the hotel dispenser or convenience store)
  - Ice packs (if you have a refrigerator with a freezer in your hotel room, chill them overnight)
  - A car refrigerator is optional (be aware that effective car fridges are very large and much more expensive than the standard cooler)

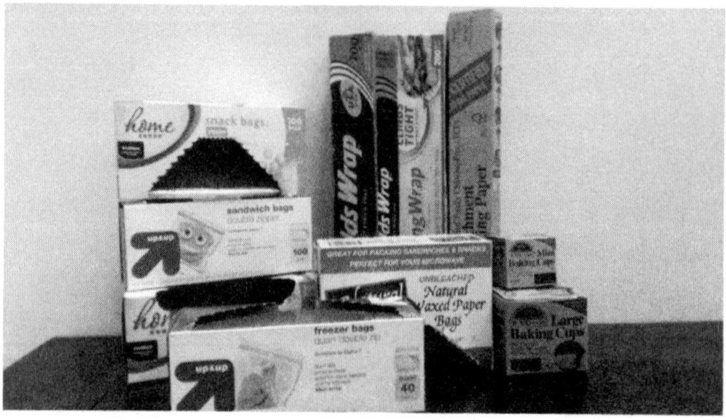

July 17, 2014

Regarding:
Name
DOB: MM/DD/Year

To whom it may concern,

Name is under my care for a health condition requiring strict adherence to the Specific Carbohydrate Diet. This diet is therapeutic treatment for a medical condition, so adherence is essential at all times. Due to the significant food restrictions that this diet requires, Name must carry and consume only carefully selected commercial and homemade foods.

Please allow Name to carry food onto planes and into theaters, restaurants and any other areas so s/he can be with friends and family but not compromise his/her strict dietary regimen.

Sincerely,

David Suskind, M.D.
Associate Professor of Pediatrics
Division of Gastroenterology
Seattle Children's Hospital
University of Washington

An example of an SCD letter from your doctor, giving permission to carry your own food.

Runny noses, coughs, and colds

Over-the-counter medications can contain fillers and additives that are not SCD-compatible or tested, so many SCD families try to manage without them. Using rubbing creams like Vicks, nasal spray, and microwavable heat packs can help relieve cold symptoms for older children and adolescents. Using a Neti pot can also be helpful to relieve congestion. I have used acetaminophen rectally for younger children and the oral form for those who can swallow pills without any problems thus far.

While fighting a cold, many individuals find it helpful to revert to Stage 1 of the SCD to ease digestion and support the immune system. It is important to make sure enough calories and liquids are being ingested to ensure hydration. Increase the intake of liquids and liquefied food: Chicken broth, yogurt smoothies, mashed cooked veggies, chicken pancakes, homemade lemonade, diluted juice, tea, and homemade gelatin desserts (not commercial Jell-O) are all good options.

Constipation

- **Eat two to three prunes per day.** Drink orange juice in the morning.

- **Significantly increase daily liquid intake.**

- **Keep SCD-compatible prune juice (made with no additives) in the house.** Depending on the degree of constipation and your child's age and size, between ¼ cup to ½ cup once or twice a day can help keep bowel movements regular and soft. Often parents will titrate the dose up or down to achieve the desired results.

- **Ensuring enough fiber in the diet is important.** The general recommendation is that 5 plus an individual's age is equal to the number of grams of fiber a person needs per day, up to a maximum of about 25 grams daily. For example, a 9-year-old child would need approximately 14 grams of fiber per day.

- **I have also used polyethylene glycol or Miralax with success** in constipated patients on the SCD.

SCD and Family Gatherings and Holidays

Holidays and family gatherings can be difficult. Empowering your child and yourself is crucial to avoid slip-ups in the diet. But even when people are empowered, it can be hard. As a diabetic child, I remember the enormous numbers of cakes and pies around our house during the holidays. I also recall that family and friends would bring over sugar-free foods for me and lay them out on the table, well-marked and very conspicuous. Although I am sure I never mentioned it to my parents, it did annoy me—to the point that I went out of my way to eat the sugar-laden foods instead.

Empowerment is important, but having a sense of ownership for the individual on the SCD is key to its success. Make being on the SCD as least intrusive as possible, especially during holidays and major social gatherings. Talk with your child prior to the event and make a game plan to make the experience fun, easy, and nonintrusive, and not a potential source of embarrassment or shame. There are many ways to do this!

- **First, make sure that as many "shared" foods as possible are available.** Remember that the vast majority of foods are SCD-safe and are delicious whether you are on the diet or not. A great example is the beautiful turkey on the cover of Ramad Prasad's *Recipes for the Specific Carbohydrate Diet* cookbook—it would make anyone salivate.

- **Second, stop, or as my mother would say, "shut down" any friend or family who tries to tempt you or your child away from the SCD.** Be proactive and proud.

- **Third, for food items that are distinctly SCD, make sure you and your child know where they are and how to serve and integrate them into the meals.**

- **And finally, the most important thing to remember about family gatherings and holidays is to have fun and be happy.** Although this may seem simplistic or even naïve, it is good to remember why we are celebrating and to be thankful for what we have.

Diet Problems

If it seems like the diet is not working and symptoms have not improved, check these potential problem areas:

1. **Does your child truly want to be on the diet?** There needs to be full buy-in from your child. If they are not actively participating and engaged, they may be SCD-compliant at home but not elsewhere. If your child isn't ready to be on the SCD, don't force the subject, as this will often backfire. Instead, find another appropriate therapy, with the knowledge that they may come back to it in the future.

2. **Check if the diet is balanced, and talk with your dietician.** Although the SCD brings down inflammation, too much of any one food item may cause a problem. A common issue is that a child will like one or two items so much that they will depend on this item excessively. I had one young lady who loved LaraBars. She ate them at breakfast, lunch, and dinner. All of her inflammatory markers, which had been markedly elevated prior to the SCD, normalized, yet her symptoms remained. After consultation, she significantly decreased her LaraBar intake and her symptoms disappeared. Other common excessively eaten foods include honey and sweets, fruits and juices, nut flours, and yogurt. Despite it's being a bit of a cliché, *variety is the spice of life*. This is especially true for diet and nutrition.

3. **Is your child ingesting hidden additives in foods and supplements?** Although the majority of the food eaten on the SCD consists of whole foods and not premade, processed foods, hidden additives can still be lurking—along with its tolls. Possible offenders may include "natural" store-bought chicken that is sometimes presoaked in a sugar-salt solution; "plain" steamed veggies at a restaurant can have a starch coating; tomato juice can contain added sugar; and prepacked veggies like baby carrots may have been prewashed in chlorine or other disinfecting solution. Additives can also sneak into the diet through supplements and vitamins.

4. **Are you adding advanced foods too quickly?** Some children may take longer to improve, and their SCD advancement needs to be tailored to each individual.

5. **Symptoms seen in IBD (such as abdominal pain, diarrhea, and fatigue) can be caused by other illnesses as well.** For example, abdominal pain is frequently a symptom of constipation, diarrhea is a sign of fructose intolerance, and fatigue is omnipresent in mononucleosis—these are all common issues during childhood and adolescence. Talk to your physician, who can help fully evaluate your child.

6. Finally, if the SCD is being strictly followed and no other problems are identified that could be affecting the efficacy of the diet, **it may be that dietary measures simply will not work for your child.** This may obviously be a difficult disappointment, but the end result of any therapy, be it medication or diet, is to make your son or daughter healthy, happy, and able to do all of the things that they want. If a therapy doesn't work, no matter how much we are invested in it, we need to find another.

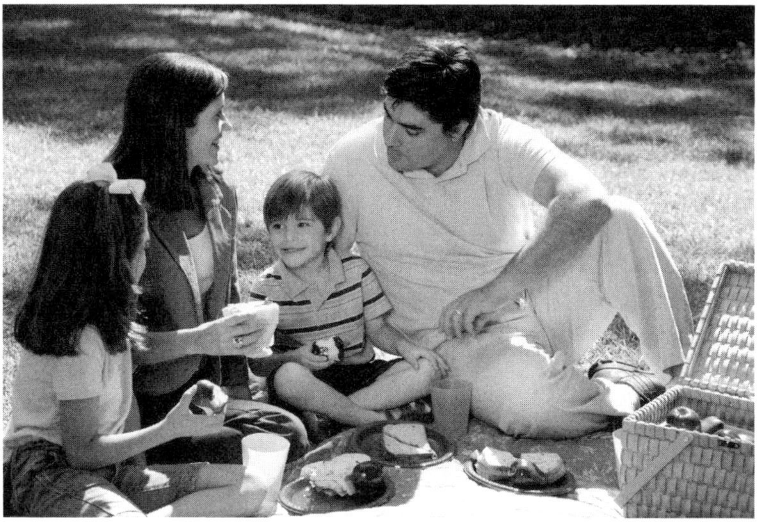

SCD and Cooking Resources

It can be difficult to know what resources are available and more importantly, how reliable they are. At the time of this book's printing, here are some of the best current SCD websites and references, as well as cooking resources.

SCD websites

- www.breakingtheviciouscycle.info
- www.eatingscd.com
- www.lucyskitchenshop.com
- www.pecanbread.com
- www.scdforlife.com
- www.scdiet.org
- www.scdwiki.com
- www.nomorecrohns.com
- www.scdrecipe.com

SCD online communities

- www.pecanbread.com/p/local1.html
  (index of local groups)

- https://www.facebook.com/groups/SCDFamilies/

- https://groups.yahoo.com/neo/groups/BTVC-SCD/info

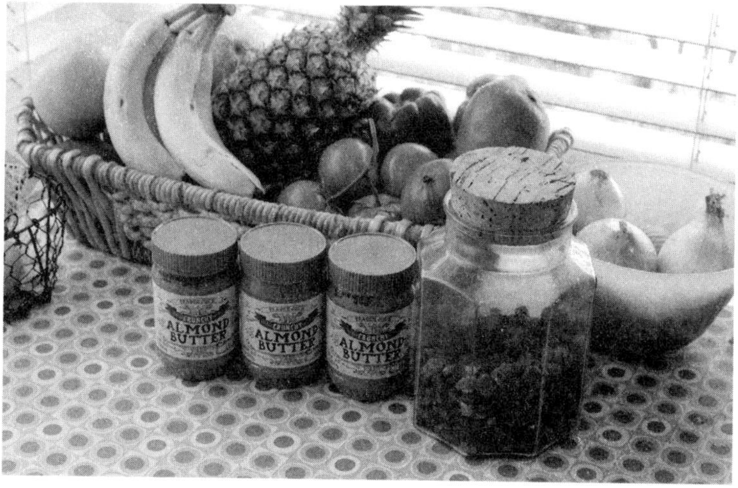

SCD-specific cookbooks

- ***Breaking the Vicious Cycle: Intestinal Health Through Diet***
  Elaine Gloria Gottschall, 1994, The Kirkton Press.

- ***Lucy's Specific Carbohydrate Diet Cookbook*, 5th Edition**
  Lucy Rosset, 2010, Lucy's Kitchen Shop, Inc.

- ***Recipes for the Specific Carbohydrate Diet: The Grain-Free, Lactose-Free, Sugar-Free Solution to IBD, Celiac Disease, Autism, Cystic Fibrosis, and Other Health Conditions***
  Raman Prasad, 2008, Fair Winds Press.

- ***Adventures in the Family Kitchen: Original Recipes Based on the Specific Carbohydrate Diet*, 2nd Edition**
  Raman Prasad, 2004, SCD Recipe LLC.

- ***SCD with Taste and Tradition***
  Rochel Weiss, 2000, Digestive Diet Incorporated.

- ***Turtle Soup: Recipes for the Specific Carbohydrate Diet from an SCD Mom***
  Beth Spencer, 2012, Lulu.com.

- ***Two Steps Forward, One Step Back: A Journey Through Life, Ulcerative Colitis, and the Specific Carbohydrate Diet***
  Tucker Sweeney and Carol Thompson, 2011, CreateSpace.

- ***Cooking for the Specific Carbohydrate Diet: Over 100 Easy, Healthy, and Delicious Recipes That Are Sugar-Free, Gluten-Free, and Grain-Free***
  Erica Kerwien, 2013, Ulysses Press.

- **More SCD cookbooks are listed on the Breaking the Vicious Cycle's website**
  www.breakingtheviciouscycle.info/books/listing/

SCD meal planning

- **Pecanbread** (website)
  www.pecanbread.com/p/how/menu.html

Basic cooking techniques

- ***The Art of Simple Food: Notes, Lessons, and Recipes from a Delicious Revolution*** (book)
  Alice Waters, 2007, Clarkson Potter.

- ***Joy of Cooking*** (book)
  Irma S. Rombauer, Marion Rombauer Becker, and Ethan Becker; 2006; Scribner.

- ***CookWise: The Secrets of Cooking Revealed*** (book)
  Shirley O. Corriher, 2011, William Morrow Cookbooks.

- **Cook's Illustrated** (magazine and website)
  www.cooksillustrated.com

- **Teri's Kitchen's Glossary of Kitchen Techniques** (web page)
  www.teriskitchen.com/glossary-a.html

- **HealwithFood.org's Vegetable Steaming Times Chart** (web page)
  www.healwithfood.org/chart/vegetable-steaming-times.php

- **Betty Crocker's Fresh Vegetable Cooking Chart** (web page)
  www.bettycrocker.com/how-to/tipslibrary/charts-timetables-measuring/fresh-vegetable-cooking-chart

- **Traditionaloven.com's Butter Conversion Chart** (web page)
  www.traditionaloven.com/conversions_of_measures/butter_converter.html

Food safety and storage

- **Foodsafety.gov** (website)
  www.foodsafety.gov

- **Home Food Safety** (website)
  http://www.eatright.org/resources/homefoodsafety

Guidelines for freezing and storing food

- **National Center for Home Food Preservation's How Do I Freeze?** (web page)
  http://nchfp.uga.edu/how/freeze.html

- **Still Tasty: Your Ultimate Shelf Life Guide** (website)
  www.stilltasty.com

Guidelines for microwaving

- **Home Food Safety's Microwave Cooking Safety** (web page)
  www.homefoodsafety.org/cook/microwave-safety

- **USDA Food Safety and Inspection Service's Cooking Safely in the Microwave Oven** (web page)
  www.fsis.usda.gov/wps/portal/fsis/topics/food-safety-education/get-answers/food-safety-fact-sheets/appliances-and-thermometers/cooking-safely-in-the-microwave/cooking-safely-in-the-microwave-oven

Buying SCD food online

- **Wellbee's** www.wellbees.com
- **SCD Bakery** www.scdbakery.com
- **JK Gourmet** www.jkgourmet.com
- **Lucy's Kitchen Shop** www.lucyskitchenshop.com

Vitamins and probiotics

- **GI ProHealth** www.giprohealth.com/scdophilusnext.aspx
- **Freeda Vitamins** www.freedavitamins.com

Preparing SCD Food

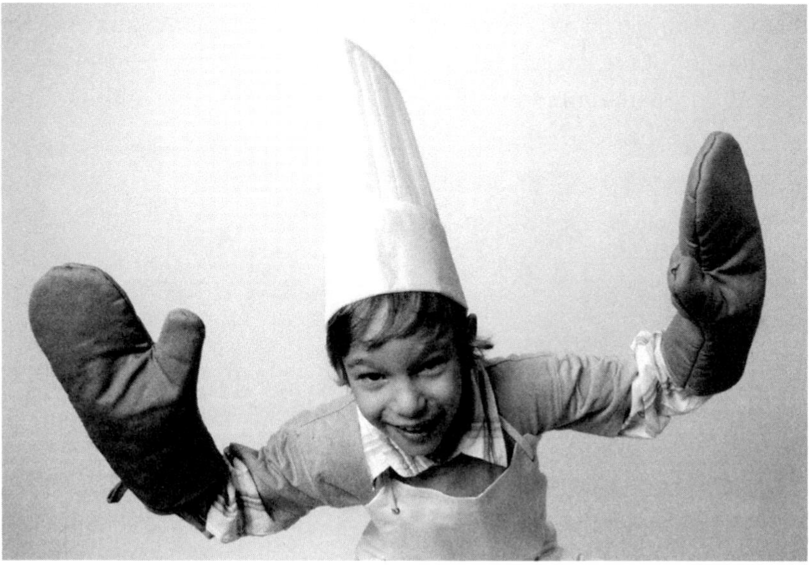

If You're New to Cooking

I don't cook ... well, occasionally I make an omelet. But I do know that it is important to have the time as well as the knowledge of how to cook from scratch. Remember that this is a learned skill that many of us already know, but many of us do not.

And if you don't, don't be discouraged! Cooking is not only learnable but it can also be fun, creative, and even relaxing. In the next chapter, we offer some helpful hints and basic cooking tips. Although learning how to cook comprehensively is beyond the scope of this book, knowing the ins and outs of the kitchen can be helpful. A huge number of cooking resources exist both online as well as within most SCD communities. Take advantage of them.

It is never to late to become a foodie!

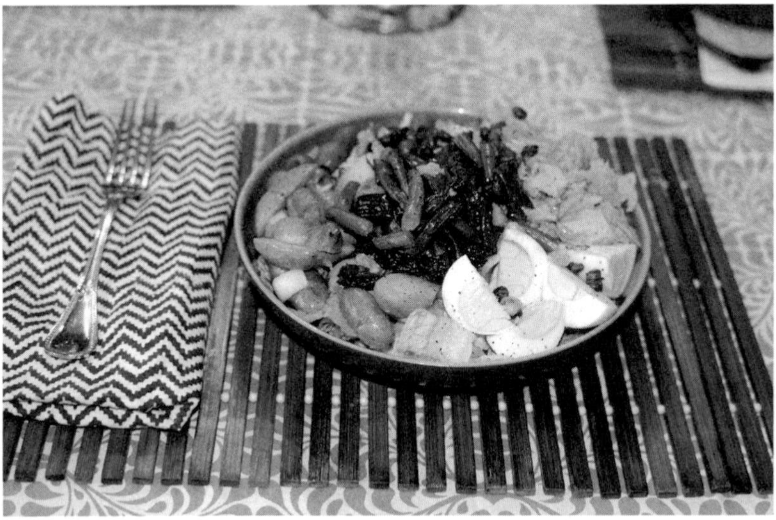

The secrets to great SCD yogurt

For many, SCD yogurt is a mainstay. It is not only cool and refreshing but it gives parents and patients a delicious and nutritious source of calories that translates into energy for activities and growth. Different people have their favorite yogurt concoctions; whether you are a purist and prefer your yogurt with just honey and fruit, or you are adventurous and like mango lassies, knowing how to make SCD yogurt is key.

It is also important for those with cow's milk allergies to know that SCD yogurt can also be made with alternative milks, including goat, almond, and coconut milks. The easiest way to make SCD yogurt is to use an electric yogurt maker. The vast majority of my patients use the Yogourmet yogurt maker. Many helpful instructions and videos exist online (including on the Pecanbread website) for making SCD yogurt.

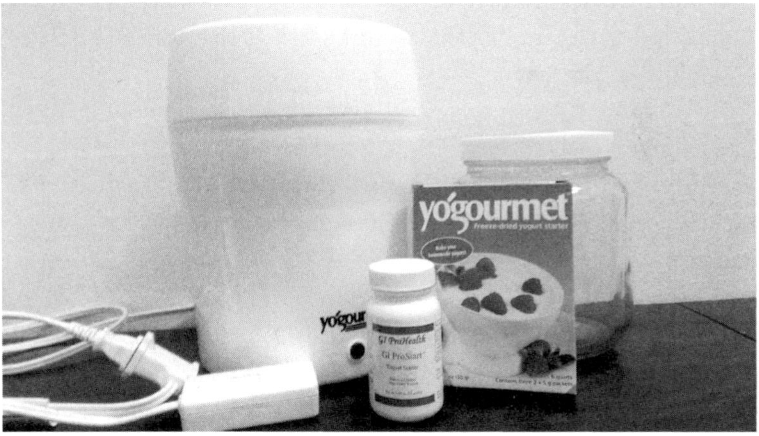

Be aware that the yogurt maker's temperature can get too hot in the summer time. Overheating beyond the recommended 100°F to 110°F can kill the good bacteria. To prevent this, purchase a plug-in dimmer switch, plug it into the yogurt maker, and adjust as needed. Always keep a small food thermometer in the water, between the jar and the yogurt maker's inner wall, so you can regularly check the temperature.

Plan ahead, since it takes about 24 hours from the time the yogurt starts until it is ready to eat—up to 16 hours of fermentation plus up to 8 hours to settle and cool in the refrigerator—so don't wait until you are out of yogurt to prepare the next batch.

Put a note on the yogurt maker marking the end time, as a visual reminder to stop heating the yogurt and to refrigerate it on time. Life is busy—you don't want to forget it for too long and waste all that hard work—and milk!

Some families even end up getting a second yogurt maker so they can make double batches at a time.

Other devices patients have used to make yogurt instead of a Yogourmet:

1. The Excalibur Food Dehydrator is a great machine that allows you to make large quantities of yogurt at a time. It also comes in handy for making SCD treats like fruit leather and meat jerky. I have been told, however, that it is a bulky machine that takes up some counter space, and it hums when operating.

2. A Crock-Pot or a slow cooker can also be used, as long as it has a 24-hour timer with temperature control. Place small jars with heated milk and starter inside. The one drawback is that it makes only small amounts at a time.

Yogurt starters

- **Never use your homemade yogurt** as a starter for a new batch! Over time the yogurt becomes more diluted and is thus less effective in breaking down lactose.

- **Dannon plain whole-milk yogurt.** This is the least expensive starter, if you can use up the entire tub before it expires. However, it is not available in every store. It is important to make sure that you are using only this specific yogurt, since similar products contain bacteria strains that are not compatible with SCD. As with any store-bought product, companies can change their ingredients, and Dannon may eventually change its bacterial strains in its plain yogurt. It is unlikely, but if this happens, you or your child can reassess such store-bought items.

- **GI ProHealth.** This is a powdered yogurt starter that must be refrigerated. It is dairy-free, so it works well with both regular milk and with almond and coconut milk. It contains *L. caseii* rather than *L. acidophilus* and is the least tart in taste. It is not available in stores, only online at GI ProHealth's website (www.giprohealth.com).

- **Yogourmet.** Use the freeze-dried yogurt starter (**NOT** the *L. casei* and *L. bifidus* kind!). Usually this is the most expensive starter and makes the tartest yogurt. This starter must be refrigerated. It is available at organic, natural foods markets like PCC and Whole Foods, or online at Lucy's Kitchen Shop (www.lucyskitchenshop.com) or on Amazon.com.

Alternatives to cow's milk

- **Goat milk.** Use gentle heat, and watch carefully.

- **Homemade almond milk or coconut milk.** You must add honey to feed the bacteria and add gelatin for texture. Can be cultured for only 12 hours. Almond and coconut are naturally lactose-free.

Coconut Milk Yogurt

Makes 2 quarts

Plan ahead, since it takes about 24 hours from the time the yogurt starts until it is ready to eat—up to 16 hours of fermentation plus up to 8 hours to settle and cool in the refrigerator—so don't wait until you are out of yogurt to prepare the next batch.

5 cups organic dried shredded coconut (unsweetened)
8 cups water
1 tablespoon plus 1 teaspoon organic powdered gelatin
1 tablespoon raw, organic, unpasteurized honey
1 to 2 teaspoons yogurt starter (See "Yogurt starters" above)

1. Place the coconut in a large pot. Add the water and bring it to a boil; lower the heat and simmer for 5 minutes. Remove the pot from the heat and let the mixture cool to room temperature, stirring occasionally.

2. Using a food processor or a blender (a heavy-duty model such as a Vitamix works well), process the coconut in several batches for about 3 minutes each time. Using several layers of cheesecloth or a purchased nut milk bag (see the Note below), strain the pureed mixture into a large bowl. You should have about 8 cups of coconut milk.

3. In a separate bowl, dissolve the gelatin and honey in ½ cup of your room-temperature coconut milk. Add the yogurt starter and mix well.

4. Add the gelatin mixture into the batch of coconut milk. Stir well to combine, then pour the milk into the yogurt containers. Ferment for about 10 hours in a yogurt maker or dehydrator, keeping the temperature between 100°F and 110°F. (Fermentation time can range from 8 to 16 hours depending on your taste preference; the longer the yogurt ferments, the more tangy it will taste.)

5. Refrigerate the containers for 6 to 8 hours. The yogurt will separate, but after it has chilled a bit—but is not yet solid—you can shake it once and it will stay a smooth texture.

Note: A nut milk bag is a cloth strainer with very fine mesh that is used specifically for making certain juices, nut milks, and yogurt. Most models are reusable and are quite inexpensive. They're much easier to handle than pieces of cheesecloth (though cheesecloth will definitely get the job done), so consider purchasing a supply of these for your convenience.

Food Safety Tips

Whether you are a seasoned cook or a relative newbie in the kitchen, food safety and sanitation are important to keep a sensitive tummy from getting more upset—or worse.

Here are some basic tips:

- **Always wash your hands with hot, soapy water before and after preparing food.** Also wash as you go, and use towels or sponges for different purposes: one for drying your clean hands and tools, and another for wiping countertops and such.

- **Clean your cutting surfaces and tools after cutting raw meat, poultry, and fish.** In their raw state, these foods frequently contain bacteria that are rendered harmless by cooking. Thoroughly wash all cutting surfaces, knives, and other tools in hot, soapy water before preparing other foods.

- **Pay close attention to refrigeration and chilling methods.** After you have cooked food, promptly chill it in the refrigerator or freezer, leaving the covers off the containers at first to allow the food to chill more quickly. If you have a large quantity of hot soup, stew, or braised meat, a good method for quick cooling is to set the bowl or cooking pot into a larger bowl of ice water. Stir it occasionally; the cold water quickly brings down the temperature of the food (add more ice as needed). Then you can package it in smaller quantities to refrigerate or freeze.

  The main thing to remember is that bacteria thrive between 40°F and 140°F, so do what it takes to get your food out of that temperature range as quickly as possible.

- **Wash produce properly, even if you're going to peel it.** Harmful bacteria and other nasties (including salmonella, listeria, and *E. coli*) may lurk on the outside of fruits and vegetables, including melons and spinach. Bacteria on the surface of, say, a melon, can easily be transferred into its interior by a knife slicing into it. Wash produce in very cold running tap water or distilled water; no soap or detergent is needed. And no need to purchase those expensive veggie washes either—although they are effective, cold, clean running water works nearly as well.

- **Never store raw garlic in oil at room temperature.** Even in the refrigerator this is chancy, as sulfurous compounds in garlic provide ideal conditions for breeding botulism, the most deadly natural toxin known to humans. However, garlic can be safely stored in vinegar (not balsamic) if refrigerated; the high acid content of the vinegar prevents the formation of botulism.

- **When it comes to canning green beans and other low-acid veggies, pay close attention to established canning standards** and do not try to shortcut any steps.

- **Refrain from washing raw meat, poultry, or eggs,** in spite of what you may have heard in the past. Washing these foods can spread bacteria to sinks, faucet handles, countertops, and other kitchen surfaces. A better way to deal with potential contamination is to make sure you wash your work surfaces and tools after handling these products, and to cook the foods well.

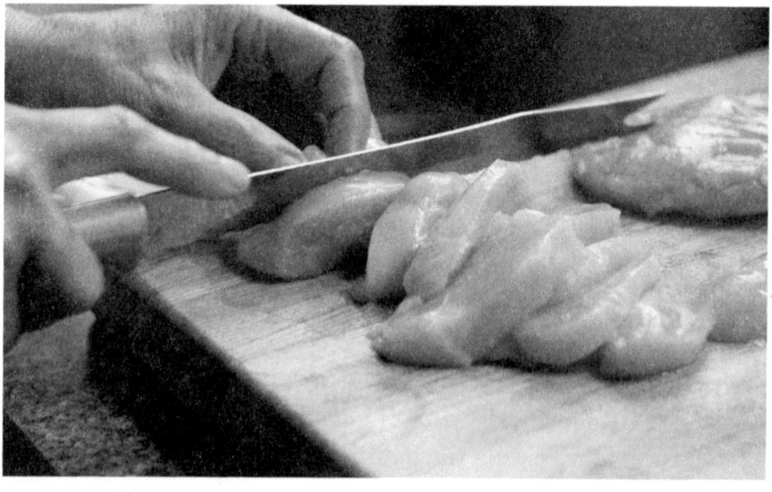

- **Don't put cooked meat back on a plate that held raw meat or the marinade** in which it was standing. This can result in cross-contamination. Always use separate dishes for raw and cooked flesh foods.

- **Reusing raw marinade on cooked foods is a no-no,** since germs and bacteria from the raw meat may still be lurking there. If you want to reuse the marinade, heat it to a boil, then use it immediately.

- **Uncooked eggs can be a problem.** Although salmonella is nowadays actually very rare in commercial egg production, it can still turn up occasionally. If you want to be extra safe, avoid eating products with raw eggs, such as Caesar salad dressing made with raw eggs, and (sorry, cookie-dough lovers!) cookie dough.

- **When you freeze foods, be sure to write the date on the package** so you'll know whether to use or discard the food. (See the link below for some guidelines on how long to keep frozen foods.)

- **If in doubt, throw it out.** Leftovers gone bad don't always smell that way—it's better to be safe than sorry. For reliable information on food storage times, see the Foodsafety.gov website: www.foodsafety.gov/keep/charts/storagetimes.html, as well as the Still Tasty: Your Ultimate Shelf Life Guide website: www.stilltasty.com.

Preparing Foods in Advance and Other Kitchen Tips

There is no denying that successfully following the SCD takes commitment, time, and advance planning. But life can be a lot easier if you prepare certain food ingredients in advance; then you can pull out these items on busier weeknights when you don't have as much time to assemble everything from scratch. Also, when your child's cravings and hunger hit, there will be far less temptation to indulge in SCD-illegal foods.

Here are some suggestions for getting—and staying—organized in the kitchen:

1. **Each week, create a menu for the following week**, make a shopping list, and get all of the groceries you will need before the weekend. Use the weekend for cooking. (See pages 50–60 in "Meal Planning.")

2. **Try to think ahead about your meal preparation.** One of the most difficult parts is remembering to take frozen meat out of the freezer and thaw it in time for meals!

3. **Use prepared, ready-to-use staples** such as frozen vegetables and deboned chicken breasts (but always make sure they contain no additives or other SCD-illegal ingredients).

4. **Make and freeze stocks and broths ahead of time.** These concoctions are the basis of many dishes, adding flavor and nutrition; homemade broths are also a major component of Stage 1 of the SCD. Freeze in convenient sizes so you don't have to thaw more than you need at one time.

5. **Have SCD-legal cans of chicken, tuna, and salmon on hand,** as well as eggs and cheese—for emergencies as well as for a quick meal at the end of a long, busy day.

6. **Always have SCD yogurt available.** Since making the yogurt takes about 24 hours from start to finish, don't wait until you are out of yogurt to make the next batch (see page 87 in "The Secrets to Great SCD Yogurt").

7. **Always have nut butters, nuts, seeds, and dried fruit on hand for snacks and outings.** These are quick, filling, and highly portable.

8. **Make and freeze marinades ahead of time in zipper-lock storage bags.** Place the frozen bags in the fridge overnight to thaw in time for an evening grill the next day. Do this over the weekend or whenever you have some free time.

9. **Freeze food in individual portions.** It makes for easy, fast thawing and allows for a varied menu on the fly.

10. **Make extra batches of SCD-legal Italian-style tomato sauce, barbecue sauce, and ketchup so you have plenty on hand.**

11. **Slow-cook a large beef roast, then slice and freeze it along with its pan juices for serving on busy nights.**

12. **A Crock-Pot or a slow cooker is a wonderful time-saver** and is great for making delicious soups, stews, braised meats, and cooked applesauce.

13. **One-pot meals, soups, and stews, frozen in single portions, are great time-savers and are very versatile.** It's easy to freeze single meals in Pyrex or ovenproof glass dishes for later thawing and heating at home or in a microwave oven at work or school.

14. **Prepare fresh-herb ice cubes for instant thawing and seasoning.** Instead of using dried herbs, which often don't have very good flavor or aroma, freeze fresh herbs such as basil, dill, parsley, rosemary, sage, savory, tarragon, and thyme. Chop the herbs finely, mix them into a paste using ⅓ cup of olive oil or cooled, melted SCD-legal butter to every 2 cups of herbs, and then freeze the resulting mixture in ice cube trays. To use, simply pop out however many cubes you need into a strainer and let the oil melt away, or just drop them still frozen into sauces or soups.

15. **Mix triple batches of dough for cookies, crackers, or pizza. They go fast!** Pizza and cracker dough can be shaped as a flat disc, wrapped

in parchment paper first, and then covered in plastic wrap for freezing. To bake, thaw and roll out or pat the disc of dough flat onto a large, oiled Pyrex or ovenproof glass baking dish or a parchment-paper–lined baking sheet.

16. **The SCD calls for a lot of baking: breads, crackers, muffins, cookies, etc.** High-quality parchment paper and muffin paper cups are helpful. The If You Care brand of parchment paper and muffin cups works great with sticky almond and coconut flours. For cookies, Silpat brand silicone baking mats work well.

17. **As soon as you get them home, preprep your fruits and veggies.** Wash, trim, cut, and place them in zipper-lock storage bags for both the refrigerator and freezer. This way the work is done and all you have to do is grab them for cooking and snacks. It also reduces food waste from forgotten or tucked-away produce.

18. **Have cut-up, prepared vegetables and fruits ready and waiting in the refrigerator at all times,** so when your child is looking for a snack, there is a selection available without extra hassle and fuss.

19. **Clean as you go.** Don't leave all of the mess for last, or it will be overwhelming!

20. **Invest in a small but efficient collection of kitchen gadgets.** Nothing is more frustrating than not having the right tool for the job at the time. Keep your knives sharpened, and have at the ready essentials such as a large, good-quality cutting board, a yogurt maker, food processor, garlic press, cheese slicer, whisk, and other items.

21. **Canning and drying your own fruit and vegetables,** especially when they are in season and at their most flavorful and economical, can be a godsend on the SCD.

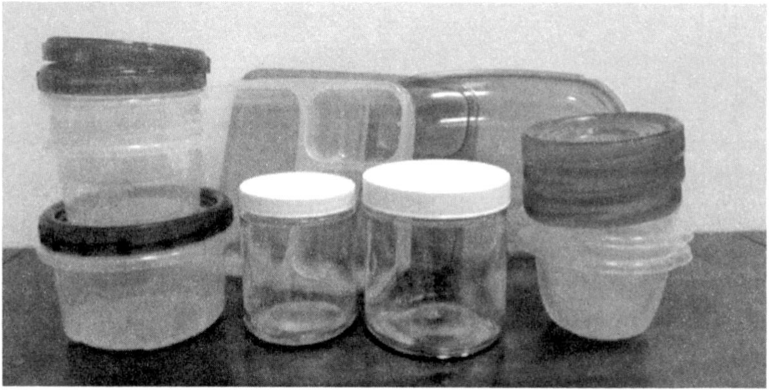

22. **Keep a collection on hand of different sizes and shapes of Pyrex or glass ovenproof dishes with covers,** other glass and plastic food containers, and zipper-lock storage bags for storing and freezing food. Sandwich bags, mini snack bags, paper wraps, and spill-proof containers as well as a variety of lunch boxes, thermoses for hot and cold items, and bottles for water or diluted juice are important. All of these items ensure that bagging lunches or packing food for an outing or travel doesn't become a reason for stress.

23. **If you are just not comfortable with cooking or don't have enough time, get help.** Take a cooking class (don't be afraid to let the instructor know of your special needs), or enlist the help of friends, neighbors, or the larger SCD community. Or, if you can afford it, hire a personal chef.

24. **If you have access to a professional, local restaurant supply store, take advantage of it.** They frequently have much better prices on items like muffin cups, or have supplies in bulk, or carry items that you would never normally find in other places.

25. **Ask around.** Hundreds of other SCD families are on this same journey as you and have developed their own tricks and techniques. Connect with them and learn something new ... and they will also learn from you!

Basic Cooking Techniques

If you are a parent of an SCD child and are new to cooking or have not done much of it before, you are probably feeling completely overwhelmed. Suddenly you may be faced with spending a lot more time planning meals, shopping, and cooking. You may also see a number of terms in the recipe section of this book and not be quite sure what they mean.

Luckily, help is at hand—hundreds of great resources on every aspect of cooking, thousands of different cookbooks, and millions of recipes exist on the Internet and at booksellers. Thanks to a burgeoning American interest in food and cooking, an entire world of cuisines is now available at our fingertips—as are many diverse ingredients that were relatively unknown or hard to find even just a decade ago. Check pages 83–84 in "Cooking Resources" for some of the most popular and reputable sources.

To get you started, here is a rundown of basic cooking techniques, what they mean, and their pros and cons:

Boiling

While you can certainly cook many foods (vegetables and even meats) by boiling them, it's not the method of choice if you want the most flavor and nutrition from your food. These days, good cooks use boiling water, often salted, to cook vegetables very quickly—actually called blanching—with the goal of removing them from the water before they become waterlogged and overdone. Once blanched, your crisp-tender, brightly colored vegetables can be eaten right away, tossed into a sauté pan with a bit of oil to shine them up, or chilled for later use.

Steaming

A good, wide steamer pot or bamboo basket will soon become your best kitchen friend, because steaming is a fantastic way to cook and eat vegetables. Steam is hotter than boiling water, so veggies cook quickly—and they also get done all at the same time. Your vegetables come out of the pot au natural, giving you a lot of control over how to season or use them after that.

Steaming may also be used for fish: Throw some aromatics (onion, garlic, ginger, fresh herbs, and whole spices) into the water, and steam a fish fillet or some prawns—there's almost no way to overcook steamed fish—and drizzle with lemon butter for a wonderful entrée.

Stir-frying

When we think of stir-frying, usually the first thing that comes to mind is a wok, that very wide, shallow metal pan that originated in China. It's great if you have a wok for stir-frying, but a large sauté pan (12 inches is a common size) is a reasonable substitute. The technique of stir-frying is simply one of adding ingredients to the hot pan (usually starting with some oil or liquid), putting in the ones that take the longest to cook first and ending with the quickest-cooking ingredients, tossing or stirring everything as it cooks. Often you'll add some final seasonings or sauce to finish.

It's important with stir-frying to know how long various ingredients take to cook and to be able to wield a knife well enough to cut even-size pieces. Because stir-frying cooks food so quickly, it is also important to have all of your ingredients already cut up and ready to go before you start heating the pan. Having said that, it seems like almost anything that comes from a stir-fry recipe tastes delicious...

Sautéing

Sautéing is, in a way, the French version of stir-frying. A small amount of oil is put into a wide skillet or sauté pan and set over medium to medium-high heat. The foods—meats, fish, poultry, or vegetables—cook fairly quickly as they are tossed (probably not with the vigor of stir-frying in a wok) over the direct heat. Often sautéing produces food that is slightly browned or caramelized, giving extra flavor and dimension to just about anything!

Stewing

Almost all of us know firsthand what a stew is: a combination of meat, vegetables, and seasonings in a sauce or broth that is eaten as a hearty, stand-alone dish. The key to successful stewing is to choose the right cuts of meat, cover the solid ingredients with a generous amount of liquid, and cook them very slowly for several hours. Flavor combinations are almost endless; think of a Moroccan tagine, an Irish lamb stew, American-style beef stew, French coq-au-vin, and so on. Many of these basic formulas can be adapted to fit the SCD plan. Last, don't forget to use a Crock-Pot or a slow cooker for your stew making—there's a lot to be said for combining all your ingredients and walking away!

Braising

Braising is closely related to stewing. Generally, the cuts of meat used are the same (the cheaper, tougher, more flavorsome ones)—but braising definitely means using less liquid, keeping the pot covered, and again, cooking at a very low temperature until the luscious meat starts to fall apart. Your mom's pot roast comes under this category, as does pulled pork for barbecue. If your recipe calls for browning the meat before assembling the braise (or stew), don't be tempted to skip this step! You'll get tons of dark, caramelly flavor notes in the process.

Frying (also deep-frying)

Think of fried chicken cooking happily in a cast-iron pan on the stove, and you'll recognize the technique called pan-frying. It differs from sautéing in that more fat is used, often to effectively surround a bumpy, breaded piece of something tasty. (And of course, for SCDers, breading means not using regular grain flour but an alternative like almond flour.)

Deep-frying, of course, implies submerging the food completely in oil. And while most of us don't deep-fry food too often at home, it's a very doable process. You'll have the most success by dedicating a medium pot to deep-frying (since the oil can coat the inside of the pot and make it rather sticky) and by investing in a thermometer that attaches to the side of that pot. Temperature is critical for making deep-fried foods that cook evenly and don't retain a ton of extra oil.

Roasting

If you're not already eating oven-roasted vegetables on a regular basis, you're going to love starting! Simply cut one or more types of vegetables into even-sized pieces, then toss them in a bowl with flavorful olive oil and a sprinkle of salt and pepper. Spread them out on a cookie sheet and bake them at a pretty high temperature—385°F to 425°F is about right—until they are caramel-brown and slightly crisped. Your kids will love the way this method adds sweetness to the flavor of their favorite vegetables.

Oven-roasting is also an excellent method for cooking meat and poultry. Think of that whole, golden-brown, herb-roasted chicken; or a garlicky roasted rack of lamb or pork; or a beef standing rib roast. Find a respected cookbook that helps you choose the proper cut of meat for this (and all) methods.

Baking

Baking can refer to the way we cook many savory foods (anything from a single squash to a casserole); it implies cooking food, usually uncovered, with dry heat.

Then there's the kind of baking that we all tend to love: the kind that produces bread, pastries, cookies, and so on. Being on the SCD doesn't mean you have to give up these things completely, but it does mean that you'll be learning a new way to produce baked goods. You'll be using different types of flour (almond instead of wheat, for instance), and natural sweeteners that are not so intensely sweet, but are much more healthful. Take baking step by step, using trusted sources for your recipes and ideas.

Microwaving

Microwaving can be a big time-saver for busy families; besides reheating and defrosting, it can also be used to precook certain ingredients that are destined for the recipe you're making for dinner. Of course, microwaves have their drawbacks: they don't always cook or reheat things evenly, and they can toughen or overcook meat and certain other foods. You can best decide which tasks they're most suitable for, depending on your style of cooking.

Freezing

Freezing can be a godsend for busy SCD families, enabling them to prepare different ingredients, sauces, condiments, side dishes, and entire meals when they have more time for cooking. Then it's easy to just pull out items for lunch or dinner, thaw, heat, and eat. Single-serving portions are especially handy for quick meals. Freezing is also a great way to stock up on meat and produce when they are in season and at their most economical. Be aware that not all foods keep equally long, so be sure to write the date on all of your items. Also, food must be properly packaged to avoid ice crystals and thus freezer burn, which changes texture and hastens deterioration. See the Resources section in this book on page 84 for freezing guidelines.

Making Vegetables More Appealing to Children

Do you have young, fussy eaters (or older adult ones) in the house who won't eat their vegetables? Won't even look at them? Do they make faces at the mere mention of broccoli, asparagus, or spinach?

Most of us have childhood memories of certain foods that our parents made us eat, or traumatizing moments when we were not allowed to leave the table or have dessert unless we finished whatever ghastly pile was on our plate. Vegetables often end up on that list, which is unfortunate.

Our tastes and food preferences are strongly shaped by the eating habits of family and friends, innate preferences, and our culture's social attitudes toward different types of foods. Our lifelong diet is profoundly shaped by what we are exposed to at a young age—even in the womb.

Whereas many American children prefer potato chips to carrots, vegetables and fruits play a much larger role in the daily diets of kids in other parts of the world. A common snack for the young and old alike in France is radishes with butter and salt; in Italy pieces of raw fennel (which taste like licorice) are served for dipping in olive oil. Young Korean children are routinely given plain cooked potatoes or corn on the cob to nibble on between meals, rather than salty or sweet snacks.

Here are some ideas to tempt your kids to eat more fruits and veggies:

- **Offer raw vegetables (and fruits) with dips.** Kids love dipping things, and just about any fresh produce is more enticing if it is simply washed, cut up, and served with little bowls of dressings, dips, salsas, spreads, hummus, nut butters, even honey.

- **Make it a fun finger food.** Asparagus and green beans are delightful to eat with the fingers. And don't forget carrot and celery sticks, bell pepper strips, pea pods, cherry tomatoes, radishes, broccoli and cauliflower florets, corn on the cob, apples, pears, orange sections, cherries, and berries of all kinds.

- **Don't mix things up.** Young children often dislike their foods all mixed together, as in a casserole, but instead prefer separate, identifiable items. Take salade niçoise, that classic French salad of whole green beans, tomatoes, tuna, and hardboiled eggs served over lettuce leaves. It is often a big hit with kids because its ingredients are arranged separately and not tossed together, with dressing served on the side. They love being able to serve themselves buffet-style, which gives them the satisfaction of making their own decisions and having control.

- **Use bright or novel colors to attract and entice.** Try serving red, green, orange, and yellow bell peppers, carrots, green-and-red-striped heirloom tomatoes, purple broccoli, red-and-white-ringed slices of Chioggia beets, or the brilliantly colored stems of the Swiss chard variety known as Rainbow Brights.

- **Make it sweet.** It's no surprise that children are attracted to sweet-tasting foods. Try red bell pepper strips, beets, carrots, heirloom and Sungold cherry tomatoes, and sugar snap peas.

- **Don't cook them.** Many vegetables, such as broccoli and cauliflower, smell strong and unpleasant when cooked. Children also tend to be sensitive to certain textures. Try cooking vegetables just to the crisp-tender stage, or serving some commonly cooked vegetables raw instead.

- **Never use food as punishment—or as a bribe.** We all recall being forced to eat something nasty or not being allowed to leave the table until we had cleaned our plates. It really serves no one to use food as a weapon, and it can needlessly cement food preferences for a lifetime.

- **Offer veggies with other favorite foods**—as pizza toppings, as a sprinkling on a favorite soup or stew, or on tacos or burritos. Some children are more open to experimenting than others; have them try it, but never force the issue if they hate it.

- **Let them play with their food.** Go ahead and make those broccoli trees, cauliflower brains, potato mice, or "ants on a log"—celery sticks stuffed with peanut butter and sprinkled with raisins.

- **Keep in mind that kids' tastes change as they grow.** Just because they thought spinach was yucky once doesn't mean that they will always hate it. Offer it again at another time or prepared in a different way—they just might like it then.

- **Sweet vegetables like carrots can sometimes be a huge hit** with children if made into frozen treats and smoothies. An avocado blended with SCD yogurt and bananas or strawberries can feel like quite a treat.

- **Serve a new vegetable with a familiar one.** Kids may be more willing to try the unfamiliar veggie if they know they will like the other one, and having this option ensures that they won't leave the table hungry.

- **Roasting vegetables intensifies their flavors,** makes them soft, and also caramelizes their sugars, giving them a sweeter taste. Almost any vegetable prepared this way (tossed with oil, salt, and pepper, then cooked at high heat) tastes great!

- **Have cut-up, prepared vegetables and fruits ready and waiting in the refrigerator at all times,** so when your child is looking for a snack, there are several options available without extra hassle and fuss.

- **Most kids love bacon.** Using SCD-legal bacon, try dressing a salad with a warm bacon dressing, adding bacon bits (and nuts), or using some bacon fat when roasting or sautéing vegetables.

Getting Children More Engaged in the Kitchen

One way to get SCD children much more motivated about their diet is to involve them in the kitchen. Learning how to plan, shop for, and cook their own food helps them help themselves to be healthier, and provides great lessons that will serve them their whole lives!

Here are some ideas to engage your children in the kitchen:

- **Involve them in meal planning.** Having kids do some of their own meal planning sends a powerful message that they matter, and it gives them an opportunity to pick and choose the foods and dishes they want. It also teaches them decision-making skills and choices with their SCD lifestyle.

- **Let kids pick out their own food at the grocery store.** Whether it is selecting a cucumber or deciding if they want fish or chicken for dinner, letting kids make decisions about their food is hugely empowering for them.

- **Have them help with chopping, mixing, and pouring.** Even young children can help out in the kitchen by slicing veggies or fruit, measuring out ingredients, washing greens, mixing batter, arranging items on a tray to be baked in the oven, snipping herbs from the kitchen garden, and decorating foods. Use child-safe cutting utensils and common sense to avoid kitchen-related burns and injuries.

- **Teach them kitchen safety.** Make sure they are aware of the dangers of hot stoves, ovens, and dishes; knives, food processors, and choppers; and potential contamination of cutting surfaces and countertops from raw meat, poultry, and eggs.

- **Grow your own herbs or vegetables.** Fresh herbs perk up the taste of food immensely, and nothing delights a child more than plucking the first ripe cherry tomatoes off the vine. Children have a natural curiosity for new, nurturing experiences, and gardening—even if it is a single pot of chives on a windowsill—is a great way for kids to see where their food comes from and how it grows. It also gives them the satisfaction of knowing that they raised it themselves.

- **Have children help clean up.** One of the least exciting parts of cooking is the cleaning. It is best to clean up as you go along, so it is not so overwhelming at the end. Children can help by wiping up countertop spills or messes on the floor, loading the dishwasher, putting away clean dishes and silverware in the drawers they can reach, and other simple tasks. If they balk, you can point out that the sooner everyone can get out of the kitchen, the more time there will be for eating, reading stories, or other more fun activities!

- **Have them set the table and help out with serving.** Younger children can set out the silverware, dishes, cups, and napkins. This task might be more fun if they and their siblings have special, personal plates or cups. School-age children can help bring out the food and serve it.

- **Keep it positive and don't be a perfectionist.** When you cook with your kids, schedule enough time so you are not in too much of a hurry. Remember that they are still learning new skills, so they won't be as quick in doing things as you are—or do them as perfectly as you might. It's also very important that they not associate the kitchen and cooking with negative feelings, getting yelled at, anxiety, and stress; these associations may stay with them a lifetime.

- **Make them truly a part of the kitchen, with their own tools.** Children love to take ownership of their destiny, so provide them with a supportive environment. It might be in the form of their own apron, a recipe box with cards they can write on, child-size kitchen utensils, special kitchen towels, or colorful measuring cups and spoons.

- **Praise them.** Be sure to let your children know when they've done a great job, and thank them for it. Then enjoy your meals together!

Adding More Flavor

The SCD needn't be bland or boring. Here are simple tips to add flavor:

- **Spices come in an amazing variety—use them!** Although they can be convenient, some preground spices have less flavor and aroma than if you buy them in whole form and grind them yourself, especially if you use certain ones in larger quantities.

    - **Invest in a good-quality spice grinder**—it will save a lot of time and hassle.

    - Bottles of name-brand whole and already ground spices tend be very expensive at the supermarket. **You can frequently find those same spices at a fraction of the cost if you buy them in loose form** at an ethnic foods store, like an Asian or Indian grocery, or in the bulk section of many supermarkets.

- **Use herbs—a lot of them, and fresh, not dried, if possible.** Adding herbs in the last minute or two of cooking will add lots of flavor, zip, and spark to meals without compromising the diet—and they are good for you, too!

    - **A storage tip: When fresh herbs are in season, chop them very finely, mix them with olive oil or butter, and pour the oil-herb mixture into ice cube trays.** When the cubes are frozen, pop them out and store them in zipper-lock baggies in the freezer. These herb cubes are terrific and easy to add to soups, stews, stir-fries, or any dish where you want a blast of fresh herb flavor anytime.

    - **And if you have space, growing herbs either in your garden or in indoor pots can be a nice way of ensuring a constant supply.** It can be a fun project for you and your child as well!

- **Do not skimp on salt, pepper, olive oil, vinegar (but not balsamic), and butter.** They are delicious, natural flavor enhancers that can make any vegetable dish more appetizing.

- **When it comes to oils, there's a wealth of choices now available.** Truly good-quality olive oils, even though they may be expensive, can be worth it for their superior flavor. Certain nut oils, such as walnut and hazelnut, are also fantastic in salad dressings or even as dipping oils for vegetables.

- **If you do purchase high-quality olive or nut oils, remember that they are generally not meant to be used for sautéing or frying foods because of their low smoke points.** Instead, maximize their goodness (and your budget) by using them as "finishing oils." Drizzle a bit over any cooked vegetable, meat, poultry, fish, or other dish and enjoy.

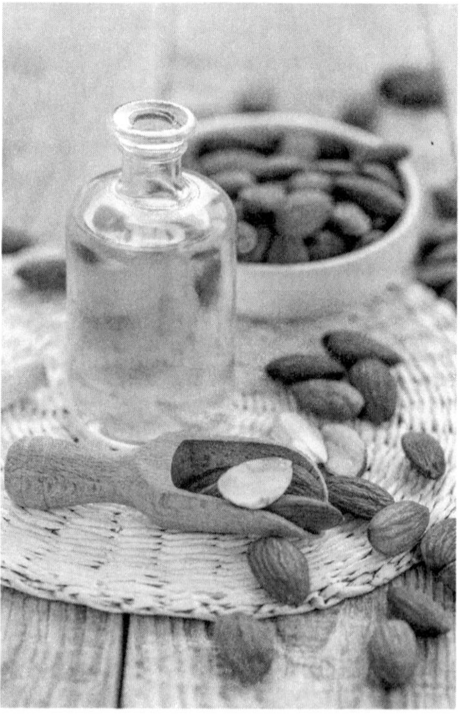

SCD Recipes

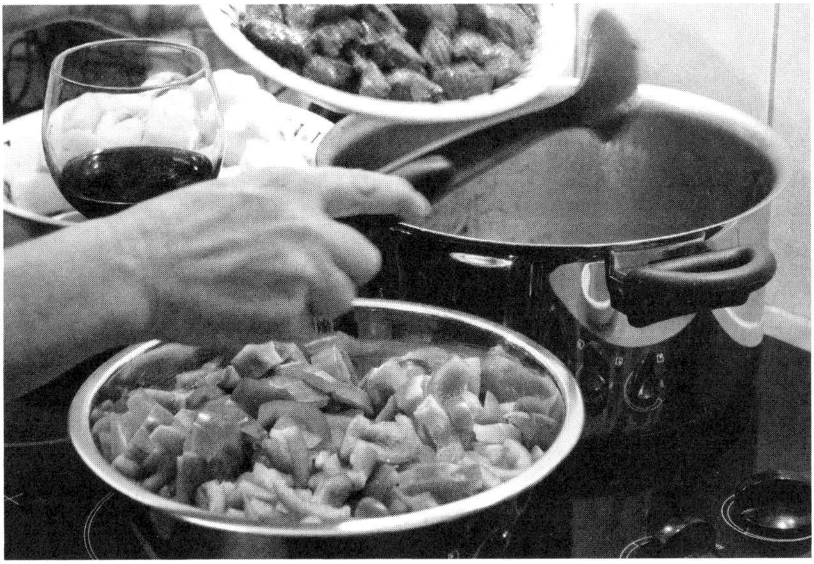

Index of Recipes

Breakfast

Snacks

Sauces

Salads

Soups

Coconut Milk Yogurt is in a separate chapter, on page 89.

Recipe Notes

Use these recipes in this book as a starting point. You'll notice that with some patience and an appreciation for whole foods, it is possible to create meals that are easy, delicious, and SCD-compatible. Try to use the freshest, natural, preferably organic ingredients possible, grown or raised without conventional pesticides and antibiotics.

Some of these recipes may seem a bit on the bland side, or they may feature flavors that you and your child may not be crazy about. Feel free to add, decrease, leave out, or vary the herbs, vegetables, and seasonings to fit your family's taste preferences and digestive tolerances.

As mentioned before, explore various world cuisines and their use of vegetables, meats, spices, herbs, and oils, as well as their cooking techniques. A number of these recipes may be adapted to incorporate these flavors (for instance, you can give the Braised Chicken Omelet an Indian flair by using cumin, curry, and ginger).

All of the ingredients in these recipes are SCD-legal. For comprehensive lists of specific foods that are legal or illegal, refer to pages 61–68 in this book and also the Breaking the Vicious Cycle website: www.breakingtheviciouscycle.info/legal/listing.

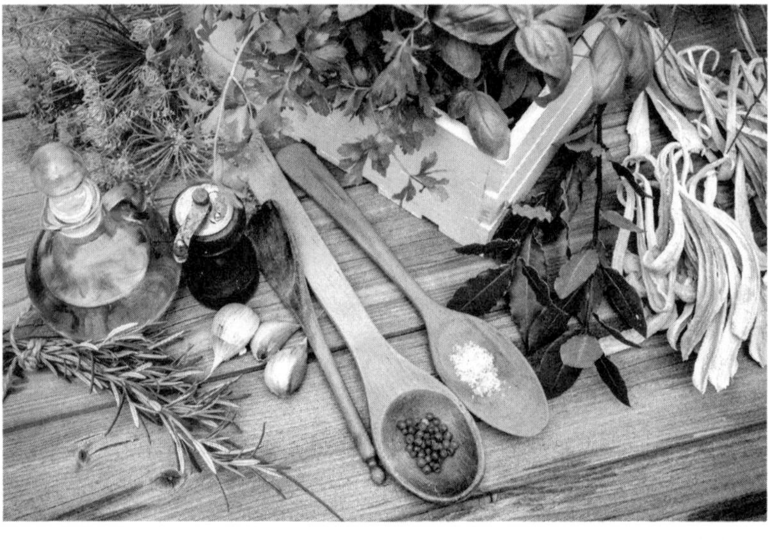

Breakfast Sausage

Makes 4 patties

These tasty meat patties are great to have on hand for immediate consumption or to use in other recipes. Cooked, they will keep for several days in the refrigerator; they also freeze well for later use. Use ground chicken or turkey instead of pork, if you prefer. Finally, to make a milder and possibly more child-friendly sausage mix, sauté the garlic, onion, and seasonings briefly before combining them with the meat.

1 pound unseasoned ground pork
¼ white onion, minced
3 cloves garlic, minced
1 tablespoon fresh oregano, or 2 teaspoons dried oregano
2 teaspoons dried red chile pepper (optional)
Salt and freshly ground black pepper
2 tablespoons untoasted sesame oil

1. In a medium bowl, combine all the ingredients except the sesame oil and let the mixture sit for 15 minutes.

2. Form the meat mixture into patties about 1 inch thick.

3. Place a sauté pan on the stove over medium-high heat. Let it heat for a few minutes; test it by sprinkling a few drops of water into the pan; they should either evaporate in a second or skitter across the pan and take just a few seconds to evaporate.

4. Add the oil and then quickly add the sausage patties. Let them brown for about 2 minutes on one side. Flip them, cover the pan, and let cook for about another 4 minutes, or until they are cooked through.

— *Travis H. Bettinson, Personal Chef, Seattle, Washington, www.junipfoods.com*

Braised Chicken Omelet

Makes 1 large omelet

You can braise the chicken leg at the time you make this omelet, or you can do it ahead of time and store the meat in the refrigerator; it will keep well for up to three days. Actually, it's very useful to braise a larger portion of chicken ahead of time, pull the meat from the bones, and have it around to use as a high-protein snack or for other dishes.

1 whole chicken leg, bone in, skin on
Salt and freshly ground pepper
About 3 tablespoons olive oil, divided
¼ white onion, minced
2 cloves garlic, chopped
2 eggs
1 tablespoon freshly grated Parmesan cheese

1. To braise the chicken leg, heat a small sauté pan over medium-high heat. Season the chicken leg with salt and pepper. When the pan is hot, add some olive oil and then quickly add the chicken leg (the oil should be hot but not smoking). Let the chicken brown for 2 minutes on one side before turning.

2. Lower the heat to medium. Add the onions and garlic to the pan; season with salt and pepper. Sauté the onion and garlic for 2 to 3 minutes, or until lightly browned. Add enough water to cover the leg three quarters of the way. Bring to a simmer and partially cover. Simmer for 45 minutes, or until the meat pulls away easily from the bone and the liquid has almost entirely reduced. Let cool; remove the meat from the bone and reserve in a container.

3. To make the omelet, whisk the two eggs in a bowl. Season to taste with salt and pepper. Heat a small sauté pan over medium heat until a drop of water evaporates on contact after 1 second. Add enough olive oil to coat the pan. Add some braised chicken meat (as much as the individual wants) to the oil and sauté for 30 seconds. Add the eggs to the pan, then swirl the pan so the egg thinly covers the bottom. Cover and cook for 1 to 2 minutes, or until the egg has set.

4. Sprinkle with Parmesan cheese and serve.

— *Travis H. Bettinson, Personal Chef, Seattle, Washington, www.junipfoods.com*

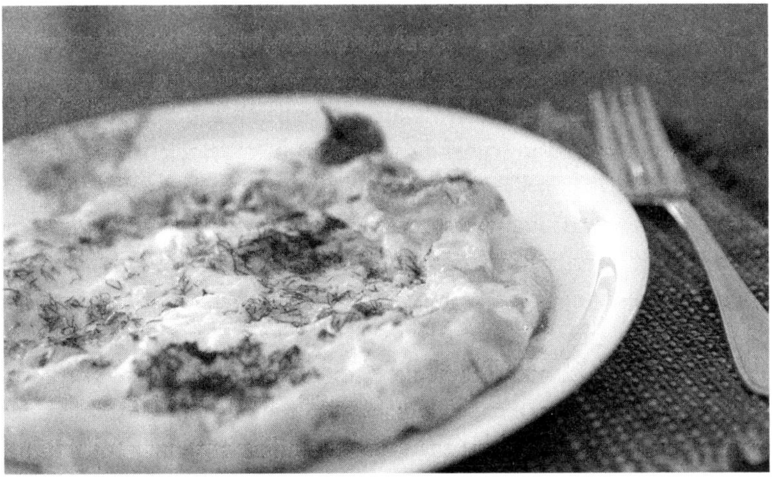

Banana-Almond Pancakes with Cinnamon

Makes 3 large pancakes

Feeds one hungry 17-year-old. Double as necessary to feed more!

1 large egg, beaten well
1 large ripe banana, mashed
2 tablespoons creamy almond butter
1 teaspoon honey (optional)
½ teaspoon cinnamon
⅛ teaspoon baking soda
Pinch of salt
Oil, for greasing the pan

1. Combine the egg, banana, almond butter, and honey until mostly smooth (small chunks of banana are okay). Add the cinnamon, baking soda, and salt.

2. Preheat a medium sauté pan (preferably nonstick) on medium heat. Lightly coat the pan with your preferred oil (we use bacon fat, but coconut oil works great, too).

3. Turn the heat down to low. Scoop about ¼ cup batter per pancake onto the pan and spread it to 2 to 3 inches in diameter. Cook until the undersides are golden brown, 2 to 5 minutes—they should release easily from the pan. Flip and cook until the second side is golden brown and cooked through. Watch the pancakes carefully, as they don't take too long to finish cooking.

4. Serve immediately. You can serve these pancakes with butter (see the chart on page 63 for more details), honey, and SCD-legal jam, jellies, and preserves (recipes are available online).

— Barbara, SCD mom from Washington

Almond-Flour Pancakes

MAKES FOUR (5-INCH) PANCAKES

¼ cup homemade almond milk (see recipe on page 123)
2 tablespoons honey
3 eggs
1 teaspoon salt
1¼ cups almond flour
1 teaspoon baking soda
Untoasted sesame oil, for frying

1. In a medium bowl, combine the almond milk, honey, eggs, and salt. Whisk together until well-blended. In a small bowl, whisk the almond flour with the baking soda.

2. Add the dry ingredients to the wet and stir until smooth.

3. Place a large skillet on the stove over medium heat. When the pan is hot, add a teaspoon or so of sesame oil to the pan and swirl it around.

4. Ladle silver dollar–size pancakes onto the skillet. Let them cook for a minute or so, or until they are golden brown on the first side. Flip with a spatula when the cakes release easily from the pan; continue cooking until golden brown and cooked through.

5. Serve immediately. You can serve these pancakes with butter (see the chart on page 63 for more details), honey, and SCD-legal jam, jellies, and preserves (recipes are available online).

— *Travis H. Bettinson, Personal Chef, Seattle, Washington, www.junipfoods.com*

Mediterranean Melon with Honey Yogurt

MAKES 2 SERVINGS

Tarragon has a subtle licorice flavor that goes beautifully with ripe cantaloupe. Of course, it may not be everyone's cup of tea, so feel free to substitute another herb if you'd like—basil and parsley are a little milder and work well, too.

3 tablespoons whole raw almonds
½ cup homemade SCD yogurt (see recipe on pages 87–90)
3 tablespoons honey
½ cantaloupe
3 tablespoons fresh tarragon, minced

1. Preheat the oven to 325°F.

2. Place the almonds on a baking sheet; bake for 10 to 12 minutes, or until they're golden brown. Let cool.

3. Combine the yogurt and honey in a bowl and whisk until smooth.

4. Cut the melon into bite-size pieces and put into a large bowl. Toss the melon and tarragon with the yogurt mixture. Top with the toasted almonds and serve.

— *Travis H. Bettinson, Personal Chef, Seattle, Washington, www.junipfoods.com*

Mushroom-and-Leek Scrambled Eggs

MAKES 2 SERVINGS

2 tablespoons olive oil
1 ounce sliced crimini mushrooms (about ⅓ cup)
1 ounce sliced leeks, just the white parts (about ¼ cup)
2 cloves garlic, slivered
Salt and freshly ground black pepper
2 eggs, beaten well

1. Place a small sauté pan on the stove over medium heat. Let it heat for a few minutes; test it by sprinkling a few drops of water into the pan; they should either evaporate in 1 second or skitter across the pan and take just a few seconds to evaporate.

2. Add the olive oil to the pan. Then add the mushrooms, leeks, garlic, salt, and pepper. Sauté for 1 to 2 minutes, or until everything is soft.

3. Add the eggs and season again with salt and pepper. Cook the eggs to your desired doneness and serve hot.

— Travis H. Bettinson, Personal Chef, Seattle, Washington, www.junipfoods.com

Savory Muffins

MAKES 12 LARGE OR 16 MEDIUM MUFFINS

Because we use natural foods in the SCD, there can and will be variations in the basic ingredients. Flavor, texture, ripeness, and other characteristics of things like cheese, herbs, veggies, and fruits will vary, and may make each batch of muffins a little bit different. This is a very forgiving recipe, though, so have fun and experiment with different options!

Our son was diagnosed with Crohn's disease at age 11. He has been on strict SCD for 5 years, symptom-free and medication-free. It takes a lot of hard work, constant preplanning, and a great dose of self-discipline, but in return it allows the freedom of wellness. We are grateful for this diet.

3 cups almond flour
½ teaspoon salt
½ teaspoon baking soda
1 teaspoon fresh chopped thyme, or ½ teaspoon dry thyme (optional)
3 eggs
4 tablespoons (½ stick) butter, melted, or ¼ cup olive oil
½ cup homemade SCD yogurt (see recipe on pages 87–90), or cooked and pureed veggies, for a dairy-free option—see the note on page 141)
½ cup shredded cheddar cheese, or ½ cup dry curd cottage cheese (omit for a dairy-free option)
¾ cup finely chopped onions
1 cup finely chopped mushrooms

spinach squash pumpkin

1. Line a muffin tin with cupcake papers. Preheat the oven to 350°F.

2. In a large bowl, mix the almond flour, salt, baking soda, and thyme. Put the eggs, melted butter (or oil), and yogurt into another bowl and mix well—a whisk works great for this job.

3. Add the wet ingredients to the dry ingredients and stir until the mixture is combined but not perfectly smooth. The overall goal here is to mix the muffin batter well but not to overmix, since that would cause the muffins to be tough. Add the cheese, onions, and mushrooms and stir to combine.

4. Scoop the batter into the muffin cups, filling them about two thirds full.

5. Bake for about 20 minutes, or until they are a light golden brown. Serve warm with extra butter alongside a soup or salad, or with school lunches or as a tasty travel snack.

Note: As with most muffins, these are best on the day they're baked. If you want to store extras, freeze them on the day of baking, then thaw as needed.

— *Tali, SCD mom from Washington*

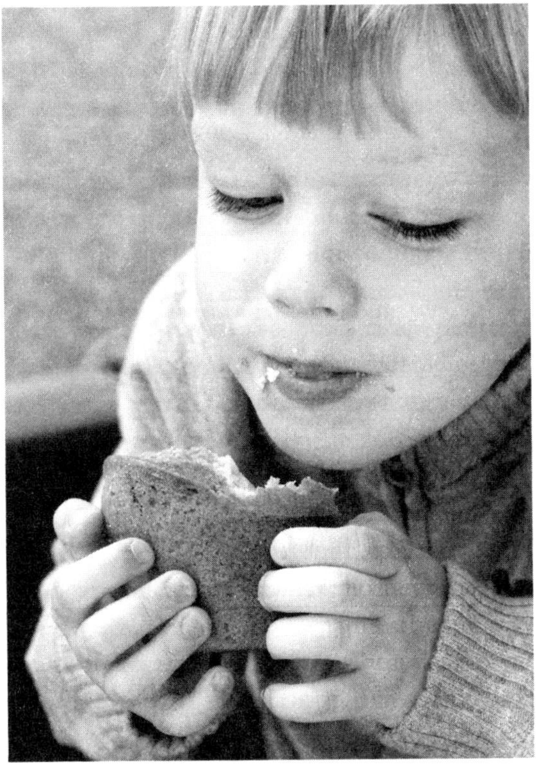

Homemade Applesauce

MAKES 4 TO 5 CUPS

Commercial applesauce, even when additive-free and SCD-legal, is made from ***fresh (uncooked)*** *apples. In the first stages of the SCD, it is advised to eat only well-cooked fruits, so this homemade applesauce is recommended over a commercial product.*

Use organic apples for this recipe, if at all possible. Conventionally grown apples are on the "Dirty Dozen" list—meaning they are extra-high in pesticide and herbicide residues, according to the Environmental Working Group, an environmental research nonprofit.

After the first week of eating plain applesauce, you may try adding a drop of honey and a small dash of cinnamon. When starting the SCD, it is important to add ingredients gradually, to help identify possible sensitivity to any specific ingredient.

8 apples of any kind and combination, preferably organic

1. Peel and core the apples. Cut them into uniform-size pieces (less than 1 inch in size) and put the pieces into a large saucepot.

2. Add a minimal amount of water to the bottom of the pot (just enough to prevent scorching, about ¼ cup). Cook on low heat until the apples release enough liquid to allow cooking on medium heat. Cook, stirring, until the apples are very soft. (If needed, add a bit more water to prevent scorching while cooking.)

3. When the apples have thoroughly broken down and are not too hot to handle, puree them, using a hand-held blender. (You may also use a food processor or a regular blender, but allow the apples to cool before pureeing them, as the hot mixture may spurt and cause burns.)

4. Refrigerate some of the applesauce for regular consumption and freeze the rest in mini-size portions for school lunch boxes.

— Travis H. Bettinson, Personal Chef, Seattle, Washington, www.junipfoods.com

Homemade Almond Milk

MAKES ABOUT 3 CUPS

Making SCD-safe, homemade almond milk is very easy and only takes a few minutes of active work. Do remember, however, that the almonds need to soak for about 8 hours—so plan accordingly. And if you use filtered water, the almond milk won't pick up any off-flavors from straight tap water.

½ cup raw almonds
6 cups water, divided

1. Soak the almonds overnight in 3 cups of the water.

2. The next day, strain off the soaking water, place the almonds in a blender (a heavy-duty, Vitamix-type blender works best) and add the remaining 3 cups of water. Blend for 2 minutes, or until the mixture is smooth and creamy.

3. Using several layers of cheesecloth or a purchased nut milk bag (see the note below), strain the pureed mixture into a large bowl. Press down on the solids to extract all of the milk. Store the almond milk in the refrigerator for up to 1 week.

   Note: A nut milk bag is a cloth strainer with very fine mesh that's used specifically for making certain juices, nut milks, and yogurt. Most models are reusable and are quite inexpensive. They're much easier to handle than pieces of cheesecloth (though cheesecloth will definitely get the job done), so consider purchasing a supply of these for your convenience.

   — *Travis H. Bettinson and Lisa Gordanier*

Easy Banana Snack

Makes 1 serving

1 or more ripe bananas
Peanut butter
Sliced almonds
Honey

Slice a banana in half lengthwise, spread peanut butter down the middle of both halves, then sprinkle with some sliced almonds and drizzle with honey. My kids call this "breakfast dessert."

— *Tari, SCD mom from Vancouver, Washington*

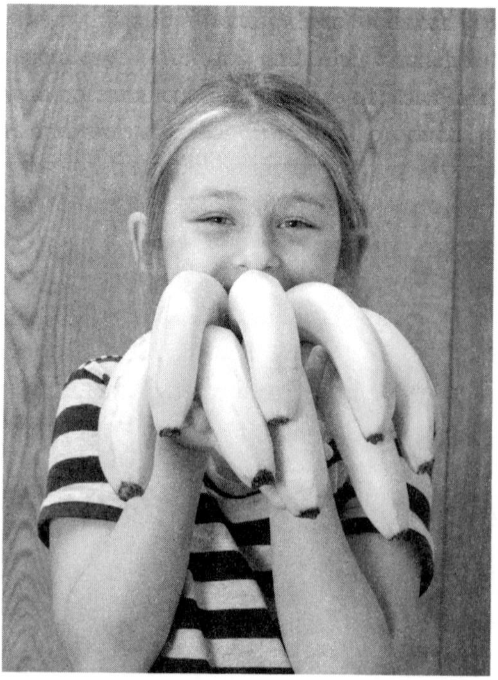

Warm Banana Pudding

MAKES 1 SERVING

2 tablespoons coconut oil
2 ripe bananas
1 egg (optional)

1. Set a medium pan on the stove over low heat. Warm the coconut oil, then mash and warm the bananas with the coconut oil. (You can always scramble an egg in for extra protein—my daughter calls it "banana scramble.")

2. Transfer the mixture to a wide-mouth thermos, and you have a quick, nourishing snack for school lunches or to take "to go."

— *Langley, SCD mom from Oregon*

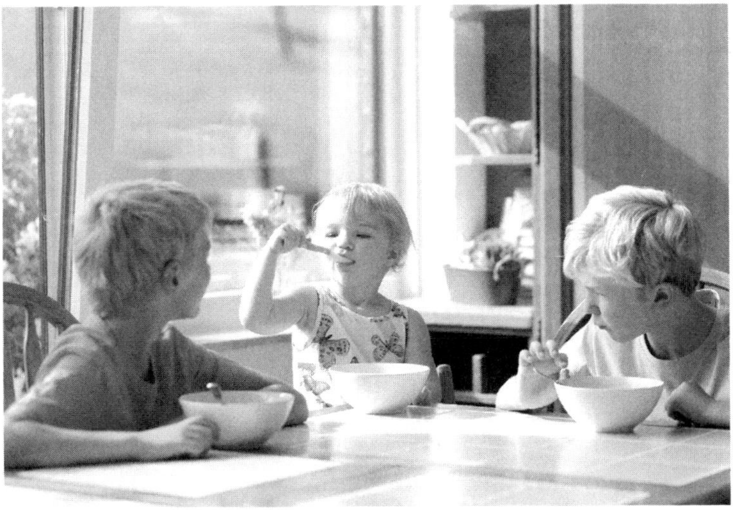

Vegetable Nuggets with Hazelnut Dip

Makes about 8 servings

Hazelnut Dip

½ cup ground roasted hazelnuts
2 tablespoons oil of your liking (except soybean)
1 cup (8 ounces) homemade SCD yogurt (see recipe on pages 87–90)
Salt and freshly ground pepper

Vegetable Nuggets

About 1 pound mixed raw vegetables (carrots, zucchini, beets, and rutabaga work well)
2 cups almond flour
Oil, for frying
2 eggs
Salt and freshly ground pepper

1. To make the hazelnut dip, mix the ground hazelnuts, oil, and yogurt. Season to taste with salt and pepper; set aside.

2. To make the nuggets, wash and peel the vegetables, then cut them into half-inch slices. Steam or boil until they're crisp-tender (you don't need to precook the zucchini). Cool them by spreading on a plate or cookie sheet lined with cloth or paper towels (this will also serve to dry the pieces, allowing the egg coating to stick better).

3. Spread the almond flour in a wide, shallow bowl. In a large sauté pan, heat several tablespoons of the oil over medium-high heat. In a separate small bowl, whisk the eggs with salt and pepper to taste.

4. Working quickly, dip the vegetables into the egg mixture and then into the almond flour. Set them carefully into the hot oil and fry, turning once, until crisp and golden. Serve with the dip.

— Morana, SCD mom from Switzerland

Bacon Bites

Makes 1 serving

These high-protein, satisfying snacks may be eaten warm or at room temperature.

Uncured, no-sugar bacon
Natural cheddar, Swiss, or other SCD-legal hard cheese

1. Fry the bacon strips until they're cooked but still a bit flexible. Set aside to cool.

2. Cut the cheese into 1-inch squares. Wrap each cheese square with a piece of bacon, cutting the strips into halves or thirds to fit the cheese. Secure with a toothpick.

— Tanya, SCD mom from Washington

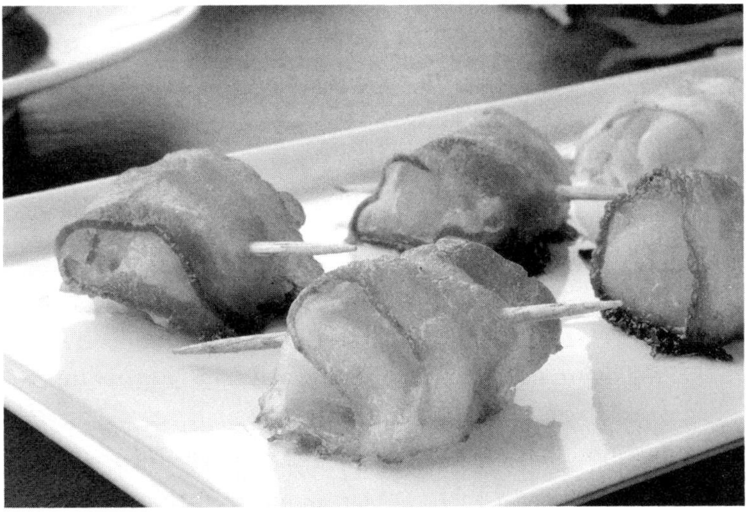

Spinach-Artichoke Dip with Mushrooms, Onions, and Roasted Red Peppers

Makes about 6 cups

This makes an addictive hot dip with pork rinds or veggies, a wonderful topping for baked salmon, or a great filling for stuffed chicken breasts. It can even be tossed with "cauliflower rice" to make a pilaf. Feel free to swap out these veggies for whatever you have, or omit things you don't like. (I use Spectrum Naturals Canola Mayonnaise, but you can make your own very easily.)

My daughter was diagnosed with ulcerative colitis at the age of 6. We have been doing SCD for over a year now and she is currently symptom-free and med-free. The biggest piece of advice I can give a new SCDer is to stick with it. The diet gets much easier the longer you do it, and the results are very motivating.

1 onion, diced
2 tablespoons butter
2 tablespoons olive oil
12 mushrooms, diced
2 garlic cloves, minced
1 bunch fresh greens (spinach, chard, kale), washed, stemmed, and finely chopped
1 (12-ounce) bag frozen artichoke hearts, thawed and finely chopped
1 roasted red bell pepper, diced
1 cup mayonnaise
1 cup Parmesan cheese, grated
1½ cups shredded provolone cheese
Salt

1. Sauté the onion in the butter and olive oil until just sweating. Add the mushrooms and cook until they're soft and have given off most of their juices. Add the garlic, stir just until you smell the garlic, then add the greens and cook until wilted.

2. Stir in the chopped artichokes and roasted red pepper, warming them briefly with the rest of the mixture. Set aside to cool.

3. Preheat the oven to 375°F.

4. Mix in the mayonnaise and most of the cheese (set aside a few tablespoons of the Parmesan and about ¼ cup provolone to sprinkle on top). Season to taste with salt. Pour into an 8-by-8-inch glass baking dish and sprinkle with the reserved cheeses. Bake for 20 to 25 minutes, or until golden brown and bubbling.

— *Cindi, SCD mom from Washington*

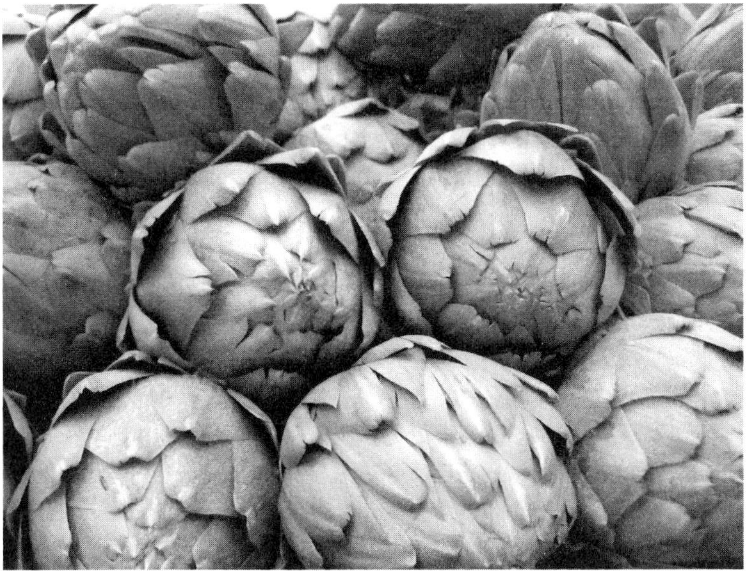

Lemon Aioli

Makes about 1½ cups

2 egg yolks
1 clove garlic, finely minced
1 small lemon, juiced
¾ cup olive oil
½ cup untoasted sesame oil
Salt

1. In a food processor, combine the egg yolks and garlic and process until smooth. Add the lemon juice and process again until well incorporated.

2. With the processor running on low speed, start drizzling the oils very slowly into the bowl. Once the mixture begins to thicken, you may increase the speed at which you add the remaining oil. (If it is added too quickly, the egg yolk will not be able to absorb it and the mixture will "break.") Continue processing until a thick and smooth consistency is achieved.

3. Season to taste with salt and more lemon juice if desired.

— *Travis H. Bettinson, Personal Chef, Seattle, Washington, www.junipfoods.com*

Sweet and Sour Sauce

MAKES ABOUT $1\frac{1}{4}$ CUPS

This sauce is especially good simmered with chicken or pork.

3 tablespoons raw honey
1 tablespoon coconut vinegar or any SCD-legal vinegar without sugar (can be purchased in some health-food stores)
3 medium tomatoes, finely chopped
Salt and freshly ground pepper

1. In a small saucepan over medium heat, heat the honey gently for few minutes. Add the vinegar and tomatoes; season to taste with salt and pepper. Simmer for 15 minutes or longer, adding a small amount of water if necessary, until the tomatoes have broken down and the sauce has thickened.

2. Taste-test and add more vinegar or honey if needed.

— *Tanya, SCD mom from Washington*

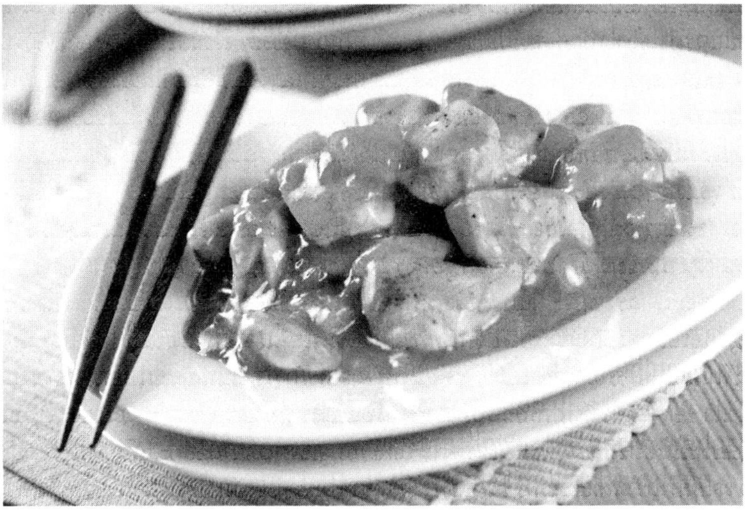

Caesar Salad

Makes 2 large salads

Feel free to dress up this salad with shrimp, grilled chicken, salmon, or other delicious ingredients such as nuts, sliced cucumber, or cherry tomatoes.

1 egg yolk
⅓ cup (1 ounce) grated Parmesan cheese
Juice of ½ lemon (about 2 tablespoons)
1 small clove garlic
1 teaspoon anchovy paste, or 1 small anchovy filet
½ cup olive oil
½ cup untoasted sesame oil
Coarsely ground black pepper
1 head romaine lettuce, chopped

1. Combine the egg yolk, Parmesan, lemon juice, garlic, and anchovy paste in a food processor or blender. Pulse until a paste forms.

2. With the motor running, slowly drizzle in the oils until the dressing thickens and emulsifies. Add ground black pepper to taste and process briefly to combine.

3. Toss the lettuce with the dressing, garnish with any extras, and serve.

— *Travis H. Bettinson, Personal Chef, Seattle, Washington, www.junipfoods.com*

Lima Bean Salad

MAKES 4 SERVINGS

1⅓ cups dry lima beans, presoaked overnight
3 tomatoes, diced
½ bunch Italian parsley, finely chopped
1 small onion, diced
3 green onions, minced
Lemon juice
Olive oil
Garlic
Cumin
Salt

1. Drain the soaking water from the lima beans. Put them in a medium pot and cover with plenty of fresh water. Simmer until soft, adding about 2 teaspoons of salt to the pot about halfway through the cooking. (Add more water if it gets low, as well.) Drain the beans and allow them to cool.

2. Mix the lima beans with the tomatoes, parsley, and onions. Season to taste with lemon juice, olive oil, garlic, cumin, and salt.

— Sue, SCD mom

Tuna Salad with Avocado "Mayonnaise" MAKES 2 SERVINGS

This recipe was born of necessity while traveling: We needed an instant lunch that didn't involve a lot of cooking, and we lacked the means to make SCD mayonnaise—so the mashed avocado became our mayonnaise!

You can fancy it up by adding cut tomatoes or cilantro, and by substituting lime for the lemon. We figure the simple version will also make good fare for backpacking. (P.S. An avocado a day has been key to my son's weight gain!)

1 (5-ounce) can tuna (in water, no broth)
1 ripe avocado
Juice of ½ lemon (1 to 2 tablespoons)
Salt and freshly ground pepper

Drain the tuna and put it into a bowl. Add the avocado and mash together. Add the lemon juice for flavor and to keep the avocado from turning brown (the color seems to hold well for 4 to 5 hours). Season to taste with salt and pepper.

—Ingrid, SCD mom from Seattle

Old-Fashioned Tuna Salad

Makes 2 servings

We like to eat this on the Parmesan-Herb Crackers made from Lucy's Specific Carbohydrate Diet Cookbook, *available from Lucy's Kitchen Shop online. You can also put this on a slice of her Parmesan-Herb Bread, sprinkle shredded Parmesan cheese on top, and brown the open-face sandwich in the toaster oven for lunch.*

1 (5-ounce) can SCD-legal water-packed tuna
¼ cup homemade mayonnaise (more if you prefer)
1 tablespoon chopped celery
½ teaspoon chopped onion (more if you prefer)
Diced hard-cooked egg (optional)
Salt and freshly ground pepper

Mix all of the ingredients, season to taste with salt and pepper, and chill.

— Stephanie, SCD mom from Indiana

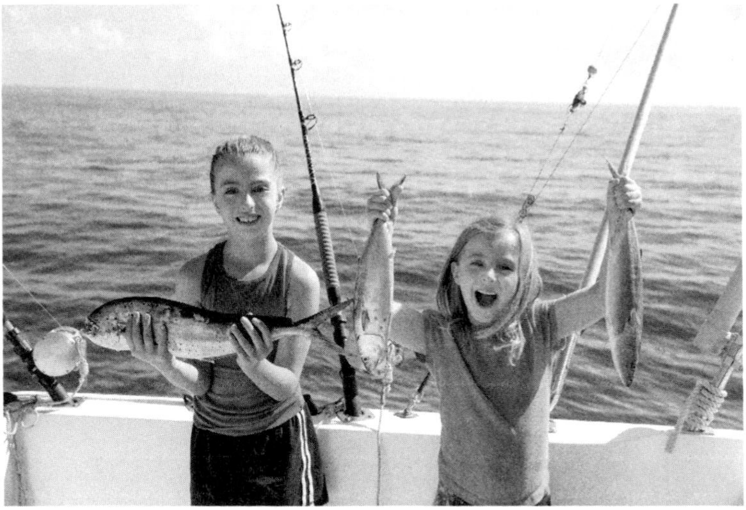

Homemade Chicken Broth

Makes about 6 cups

In making chicken broth, the backs, necks, wings, and other bony parts are very desirable, since they produce a rich, gelatinous product. (And they're cheap!) Breast pieces will yield the least flavor and nutrients.

To date there is no commercial SCD-legal chicken broth.

2 pounds chicken parts, bone in, skin on (any combination will do—see the headnote above)
1 onion, sliced
4 medium carrots, sliced
4 ribs celery, sliced
10 sprigs of fresh herbs (one kind or a mix of dill, cilantro, parsley, thyme, etc.)
Salt and freshly ground black pepper

1. Put all of the ingredients into a large (8- to 10-quart) stockpot. Fill the pot with enough cold water to cover the ingredients by 1 inch.

2. Bring to a boil, immediately reduce the heat, and skim off the grayish scum that will rise (for the first few minutes) from the surface of the water. Cover and simmer on very low heat for 2 to 3 hours, or until the vegetables and chicken are falling apart.

3. Pour everything through a fine mesh strainer, being sure to catch the stock in a large bowl below it! Press on the solids to extract all the liquid. Store the broth in the refrigerator, or freeze it in individual portions.

— Travis H. Bettinson, Personal Chef, Seattle, Washington, www.junipfoods.com

Peppery Vegetable Soup

MAKES 4 SERVINGS

Like most soups and stews, this one becomes more flavorful after a day or two in the refrigerator. It might even be a good idea to make a double batch so there's enough for the whole family!

2 medium carrots, cut into ½-inch cubes (or small rounds)
2 large shallots, diced
2 teaspoons minced fresh ginger
3 cloves garlic, minced
2 tablespoons vegetable oil
Salt
½ English cucumber, cut into ½-inch cubes (or small rounds)
Generous handful green beans, cut into ½-inch slices
2½ cups water or homemade chicken broth (see recipe on page 136)
2 tablespoons black peppercorns, freshly ground

1. Combine the carrots, shallots, ginger, garlic, vegetable oil, and salt to taste in a medium pot. Cover and place over low heat; cook for 5 to 6 minutes, stirring occasionally, until the vegetables begin to release some juices and become aromatic.

2. Add the cucumber, green beans, and a little more salt to taste. Add the water and bring to a boil. Lower the heat to a simmer and continue to cook for 7 to 10 minutes, or until the carrots and green beans are soft. Add the pepper and serve.

— Travis H. Bettinson, Personal Chef, Seattle, Washington, www.junipfoods.com

Un-Tomato Soup

MAKES 2 TO 3 SERVINGS

My daughter loves tomatoes but can't seem to tolerate them right now. As a substitute, I made this soup for her, and she loves it! You can make it thicker by adding more puree—or just by cooking it longer on the stovetop. Finely chopped cilantro makes a beautiful garnish and perks the flavor up as well.

½ cup carrot puree (see the note below)
½ cup acorn squash puree (see the note below)
4 cups chicken broth
1-inch knob ginger, peeled and grated
Salt
Cilantro, finely chopped, for garnish

1. Prepare the carrot and squash purees ahead of time.

2. Combine the broth, carrot puree, squash puree, and ginger in a medium saucepot. Add salt to taste. Simmer gently for about 15 minutes. Serve with a sprinkle of chopped cilantro on top (or substitute parsley for a non-cilantro lover).

Note: To make carrot or squash puree, first cook the vegetables until they're quite soft. Steaming, boiling, or microwaving are all good methods for this purpose. Cool slightly, then blend until smooth in a food processor or blender.

It's smart, especially when your vegetables of choice are in season (therefore abundant, relatively inexpensive, and highly nutritious) to prepare large quantities of the purees, package them in smaller amounts, and freeze them for later use.

— Langley, SCD mom from Oregon

Green Soup

MAKES 2 TO 3 SERVINGS

4 cups chicken broth
¼ cup spinach puree (see the note below)
Salt

Combine the broth and spinach puree in a medium saucepot. Bring to a low simmer; season to taste with salt.

— Langley, SCD mom from Oregon

Note: To make spinach puree from fresh spinach, start with one large bunch. Wash it well, remove the stems, and pile it in a large sauté pan over medium heat (leave some of the water clinging to the leaves). Move the leaves around in the pan; they'll wilt and cook down quickly. Let the spinach cool a bit, then puree it until very smooth in a blender or food processor.

If you're starting with frozen spinach, thaw the block completely and puree as described above. Refreeze any extra for another use.

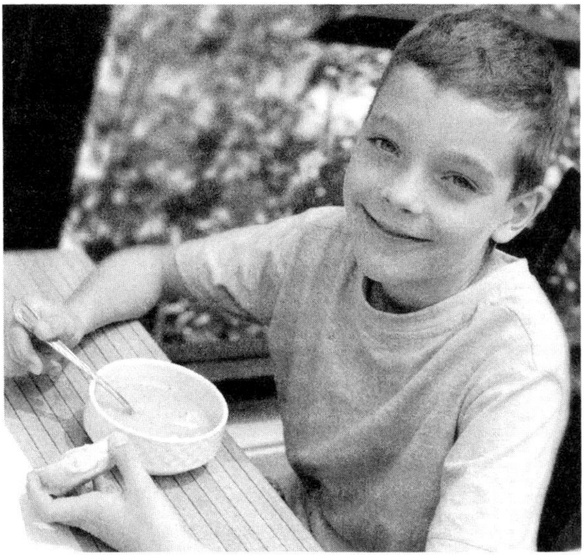

Thai Carrot Soup

MAKES 2 TO 3 SERVINGS

1 boneless, skinless chicken breast half
2 cups homemade chicken broth (see recipe on page 136)
1-inch knob ginger, peeled and cut into several chunks
3 tablespoons carrot puree (see the note below)
1 tablespoon minced cilantro
2 tablespoons coconut milk
Salt

1. In a medium saucepot set over medium-low heat, cook the chicken in the broth with the knob of ginger. Simmer gently until the chicken is cooked through. Add the carrot puree and cilantro. Simmer for several minutes more to allow the flavors to develop.

2. Remove the ginger, then process the soup in a blender or food processor until smooth (you may want to cut up the chicken breast before blending). Add the coconut milk and season to taste with salt.

— *Langley, SCD mom from Oregon*

Note: To make carrot or squash puree, first cook the vegetables until they're quite soft. Steaming, boiling, or microwaving are all good methods for this purpose. Cool slightly, then blend until smooth in a food processor or blender.

It's smart, especially when your vegetables of choice are in season (therefore abundant, relatively inexpensive, and highly nutritious) to prepare large quantities of the purees, package them in smaller amounts, and freeze them for later use.

Blended Chicken and Vegetable Soup

MAKES 2 TO 3 SERVINGS

2 cups homemade chicken broth (see recipe on page 136)
1 chicken thigh, skin removed
2 tablespoons carrot puree (see the note below)
2 tablespoons spinach puree (see the note below)
1 tablespoon acorn squash puree (see the note below)
Salt
1 tablespoon finely chopped cilantro

1. In a medium saucepot, bring the broth to a boil. Add the chicken thigh and simmer until it is fully cooked. Remove the meat from the bone, allow it to cool a bit, and then cut the meat into chunks.

2. Transfer the chicken pieces to a blender along with broth. Blend until the chicken is finely shredded, then return the mixture to the pot. Add the carrot, spinach, and squash purees, season to taste with salt, and heat thoroughly. Garnish with a sprinkle of the cilantro.

— Langley, SCD mom from Oregon

Note: To make carrot or squash puree, first cook the vegetables until they're quite soft. Steaming, boiling, or microwaving are all good methods for this purpose. Cool slightly, then blend until smooth in a food processor or blender.

To make spinach puree from fresh spinach, start with one large bunch. Wash it well, remove the stems, and pile it in a large sauté pan over medium heat (leave some of the water clinging to the leaves). Move the leaves around in the pan; they'll wilt and cook down quickly. Let the spinach cool a bit, then puree it until very smooth in a blender or food processor. If you're starting with frozen spinach, thaw the block completely and puree as described above. Refreeze any extra for another use.

It's smart, especially when your vegetables of choice are in season (therefore abundant, relatively inexpensive, and highly nutritious) to prepare large quantities of the purees, package them in smaller amounts, and freeze them for later use.

Tomato Soup

MAKES 2 SERVINGS

2 tablespoons olive oil
½ small white onion, cut into large dice
5 cloves garlic
Salt and freshly ground pepper
2 pounds (4 to 5 large) ripe fresh tomatoes, roughly chopped
1 small box (¾ ounce) fresh basil

1. Pour the oil into a stockpot; add the onion and garlic. Place the pot on the stove and turn it to low heat. Season with salt and pepper and then cover the pot. Let the onions and garlic cook for 7 to 10 minutes, stirring occasionally, until they have released some of their juices.

2. Add half of the tomatoes to the pot. Increase the heat to medium, season with a bit more salt and pepper, cover, and continue to cook for another 15 minutes.

3. Remove the pot from the stove. Cut or tear any large basil leaves, then add them to the pot, along with the rest of the tomatoes.

4. Ladle several spoonfuls of the soup into a blender and puree it until smooth. Add more until the entire soup is pureed. Add more water to the soup (or use homemade chicken broth—recipe on page 136) until you are satisfied with the consistency. Season to taste with salt and pepper and serve.

— Travis H. Bettinson, Personal Chef, Seattle, Washington, www.junipfoods.com

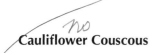

Cauliflower Couscous

Makes 2 servings

1½ pounds (1 medium head) cauliflower florets, cut into 1-inch pieces
2 tablespoons olive oil
1 cup sliced leeks
3 cloves garlic, minced
1 medium carrot, finely diced
Salt and freshly ground pepper
1 small zucchini, diced
1 cup water
2 tablespoons minced parsley
⅔ cup freshly grated Parmesan cheese

1. Place the cauliflower in a food processor. Pulse until the granules resemble couscous-size beads.

2. Place a skillet on the stove over medium heat. Add the oil, leeks, garlic, and carrot to the pan. Season with salt and pepper, then sauté them for 4 minutes, or until softened a little. Add the zucchini and sauté for another 3 minutes, or until soft.

3. Add the cauliflower and sauté for about one minute. Pour the water over the mixture, season with a bit more salt and pepper, and cook gently until the water has been absorbed and the cauliflower is soft.

4. Transfer to a serving bowl, stir in the parsley, and top with Parmesan cheese.

— Travis H. Bettinson, Personal Chef, Seattle, Washington, www.junipfoods.com

Spinach and Egg Flan

MAKES 3 FLANS

These cupcake-size individual flans make a great accompaniment to almost any meat or fish entrée. They have a gentle, mellow flavor and texture—somewhat like an expertly cooked French quiche. This version uses cooked fresh spinach, but you can easily substitute or add other vegetables such as sautéed leeks or minced onion, other greens, bits of sautéed mushrooms, or even a pinch of crabmeat.

You'll need to make the almond milk a day or so before using it in the flan; the recipe is on page 123.

2 eggs, well beaten
⅓ cup homemade almond milk
1 (10-ounce) bag fresh baby spinach
2 tablespoons freshly grated Parmesan cheese
1 teaspoon salt
1 teaspoon freshly ground pepper

1. Preheat the oven to 350°F. You'll be using a regular-size muffin or cupcake tin; if it is nonstick, you can just use it as is. If not, lightly butter 3 of the cups.

2. To prepare the spinach, bring a 4-quart pot of water to a rolling boil. Once boiling, put all of the spinach into the pot and let it boil for 10 seconds. Remove the pot from the stove, strain the spinach out into a colander, and run cold water over it until it is cool to the touch. Squeeze as much water as possible out of all of the spinach, then chop it coarsely.

3. Combine all of the ingredients in a bowl. Using a ladle or a measuring cup, fill the muffin cups about two-thirds full.

4. Place the muffin tin in a roasting pan or another deep-sided baking pan. Carefully fill the roasting pan with hot water until it comes to 2 inches from the top. Cover the larger pan with aluminum foil (allowing the egg mixture to steam) and place it in the oven. Bake for 12 to 15 minutes. Check to see if the flans have set (they will jiggle like Jell-O or not move at all if shaken). If they appear loose or liquidy in the center, let cook for several more minutes and check again.

5. Take the flans out of the oven, immediately remove the foil, and lift the muffin tin out of the roasting pan. Let the flans sit on the counter for several minutes as they set further, then serve them warm or even at room temperature. They'll keep for several days in the refrigerator; warm them gently in the microwave or oven.

— Travis H. Bettinson, Personal Chef, Seattle, Washington, www.junipfoods.com

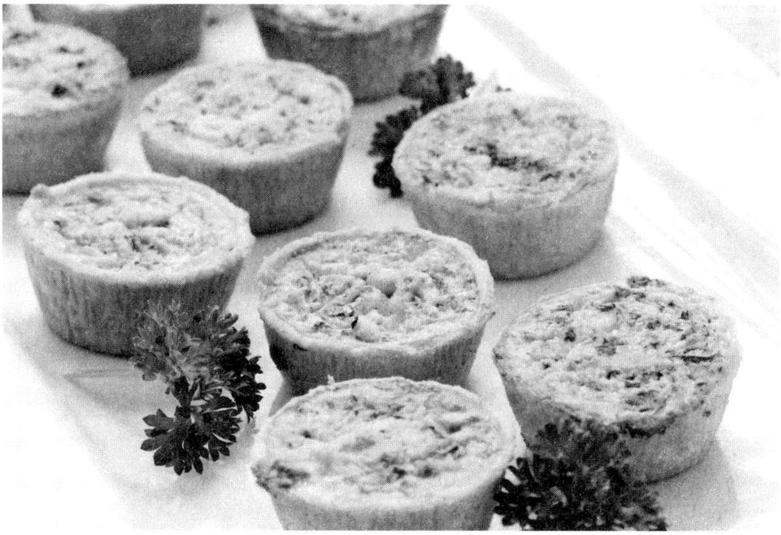

Roasted Broccoli with Sesame Oil, Ginger, and Garlic

Makes 2 servings

2 large crowns broccoli
One 3-inch section peeled ginger, grated on a Microplane grater
1 clove garlic, grated on a Microplane grater
Salt
6 tablespoons toasted sesame oil (see the note below)

1. Preheat the oven to 385°F. (To properly roast the broccoli, the temperature needs to be at least this high. If your oven runs low, increase the temperature to accommodate.)

2. Chop the broccoli into 1- to 1½-inch florets, using only the tops (save the stems for another use).

3. Combine the ginger, garlic, salt, and oil in a medium bowl and stir to combine. Add the broccoli florets and toss thoroughly so the oil mixture is evenly distributed. Let marinate for 30 minutes.

4. Distribute the broccoli evenly on a baking pan. Bake for 15 to 20 minutes, or until the broccoli florets have crisped and turned brown on the exposed surfaces.

Note: For a milder-tasting dish, use a combination of toasted sesame oil plus a more neutral oil such as untoasted sesame oil, safflower oil, or another SCD-approved cooking oil.

— Travis H. Bettinson, Personal Chef, Seattle, Washington, www.junipfoods.com

Zucchini al Limon

Makes 2 servings

This zippy vegetable side dish is fantastic with a grilled or seared steak, sliced very thin. Actually, it goes very well alongside most proteins—grilled chicken, fish, or even other vegetables.

2 medium zucchini
1 box (¾ ounce) fresh basil, sliced into thin ribbons
¼ cup olive oil
2 lemons, freshly juiced
Salt and freshly ground pepper
Parmesan cheese

1. Slice the zucchini into very fine rounds—about ⅛-inch thick—and place in a large bowl. Add the basil, olive oil, and lemon juice. Toss and season to taste with salt and pepper.

2. Use a potato peeler to shave slices of the Parmesan cheese. Place on top of the salad and serve.

— *Travis H. Bettinson, Personal Chef, Seattle, Washington, www.junipfoods.com*

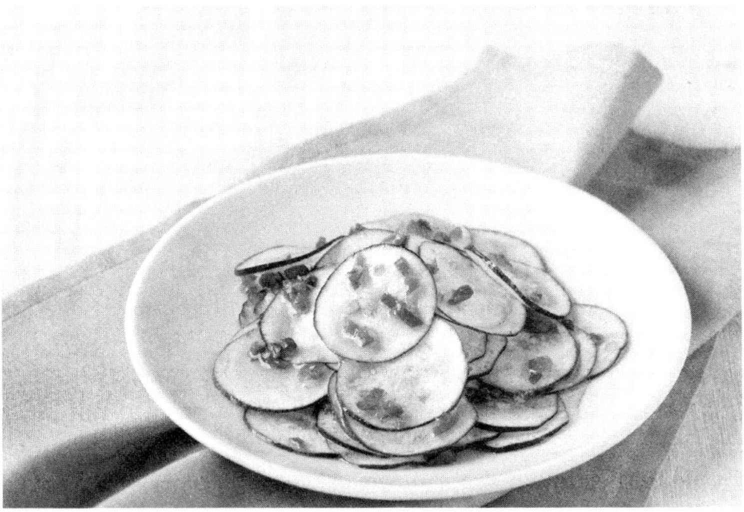

Chicken-Veggie Patties

YIELDS EIGHT (3-INCH) PATTIES

Everybody likes sausages, hamburger or chicken patties, and meat loaf, right? This recipe for SCD-legal chicken-veggie patties is basically a version of those universal favorites. Ground chicken combined with some vegetables and herbs, then fried in a healthy oil makes a satisfying addition to breakfast or as the main entree at dinner. It is incredibly versatile—meaning that you could start with a different SCD-legal meat, use different vegetables (finely minced carrots, zucchini, other greens like kale or chard), plus add different herbs and spices—all with the goal of tailoring the end product to your child's taste.

While you're getting creative, however, please aim for keeping the proportions of the patties to 1 part chicken and 2 parts cooked veggies.

2½ tablespoons olive oil, divided
½ small yellow onion, finely diced
2 cloves garlic, minced
1 teaspoon mild chili powder (organic without caking agent)
1 teaspoon fresh thyme, or ½ teaspoon dried thyme (optional)
2 teaspoons salt
½ pound fresh green beans, trimmed
1 (5-ounce) bag fresh spinach leaves, or ½ box (5 ounces) frozen spinach, thawed
8 to 10 ounces plain ground chicken meat
1 egg, beaten
Salt and freshly ground pepper

1. Heat 1 tablespoon of the oil in a medium sauté pan over medium heat; add the onion and garlic. Cook these slowly, stirring occasionally, until the onion is soft and translucent. Add the chili powder and thyme and heat for a minute or two. Set aside.

2. Cook the green beans: Fill a medium-size saucepot with water and set it over high heat; add the 2 teaspoons salt and bring to a boil. Drop the beans into the water and boil for about 5 minutes, or until they're soft but not mushy. Using a slotted spoon or a small strainer, lift the beans out of the water and put them into a bowl of cold water to stop the cooking.

3. When the beans are cool, drain them on a clean towel and then either chop them by hand until they're in very small pieces, or (easier and faster!) cut them into 2-inch lengths and whirl them in a food processor for a few seconds. Don't make them into a puree—the goal is to have them in very small pieces to blend better with the ground chicken.

4. To prepare the spinach: If you're starting with fresh spinach, use your already-hot water from the beans to blanch the leaves. Bring the water back to a boil, dump all the leaves in at once, let cook for 2 minutes, then drain well. Spread the leaves in a single layer on a cookie sheet (or on your clean countertop) to cool rapidly. Squeeze the spinach dry, then chop it coarsely; this is a job better done with a knife rather than in the food processor. (If you're using thawed frozen spinach, break up the block with your fingers and spread it onto a plate. Squeeze the water out of it, then chop it coarsely.)

5. To assemble the patties, put the ground chicken into a large bowl along with the egg, the chopped beans and spinach, and the onion mixture. Season to taste with salt and pepper. Mix well.

6. To form the patties, scoop even-size balls (2 to 3 inches in diameter and about 1½ inches thick) onto a plate. Then begin flattening and shaping the patties into discs. If the mixture is too sticky to work with, you can use a couple of tricks to make it easier: Chill the meat thoroughly; it will firm up and be easier to handle. It also helps to moisten your hands with cold water, then try the patting process again.

7. To fry the patties, heat a sauté pan with the remaining 1½ tablespoons of oil over medium to medium-high heat. Place the patties in the pan (don't overcrowd them or they'll steam rather than fry) and cook, turning once, until they're golden brown and slightly crispy on each side.

— *Lisa Gordanier*

Braised Beef with Fennel

Makes 4 servings

2 tablespoons untoasted sesame oil
2 pounds beef (chuck or shoulder roast)
1 small onion, diced
3 cloves garlic, minced
4 Roma tomatoes, roughly chopped
4 sprigs fresh thyme, or two teaspoons dried thyme leaves
1 tablespoon fennel seeds
Salt and freshly ground pepper

1. Preheat the oven to 325°F.

2. Place a medium Dutch oven over medium-high heat. Let it heat for 2 to 3 minutes, then add the oil carefully (you don't want it to splatter on your skin!). Place the meat into the pan. Take the time to brown the meat well (3 to 4 minutes on each side); this step will pay off in extra-deep flavor.

3. Remove the meat from the pan, lower the heat to medium and add the onion, garlic, tomatoes, thyme, and fennel seeds. Season to taste with salt and pepper; cook, stirring occasionally, for 4 to 5 minutes, or until soft.

4. Add the beef back to the pot (in a single layer, if possible), and add water until it comes about three-quarters of the way up the sides of the meat. Place a lid on the pot, and bring the liquid to a boil.

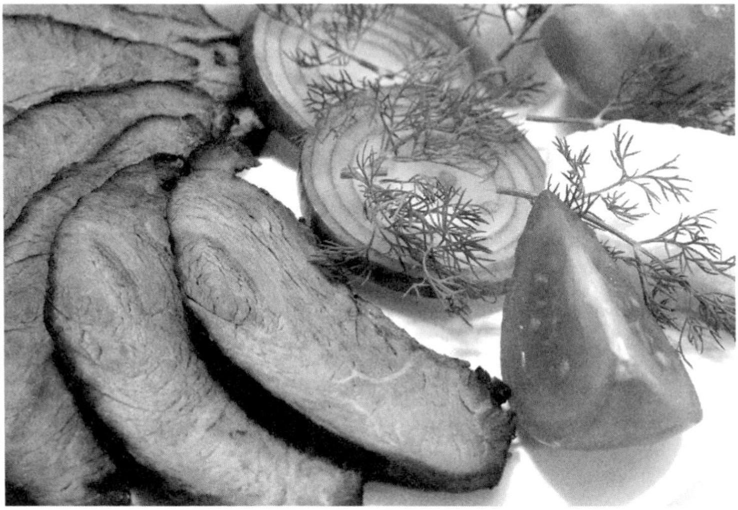

5. Place the covered pot in the oven. Let it cook for 2½ hours, checking occasionally to make sure the liquid stays at a low simmer—it should not be boiling or simmering vigorously. Lower the oven temperature as needed. It is also important to note the water level: If only one-third of the water remains, you should add warm water up to the two-thirds point.

6. Check the meat; when it pulls apart easily with a fork, it is done. If it is more resistant, leave it in the oven and check it every 30 minutes until it can be pulled apart very easily.

— *Travis H. Bettinson, Personal Chef, Seattle, Washington, www.junipfoods.com*

Biscuits with Chicken and Gravy

Makes 4 servings

Chicken

3 chicken legs, bone in

1 tablespoon salt

1 tablespoon freshly ground pepper

Biscuits

2½ cups almond flour

¼ cup butter, softened

½ teaspoon baking soda

2 eggs, beaten

1 tablespoon honey

1. Preheat the oven to 350°F.

2. Put the chicken legs, salt, and pepper in a small pan. Cover the legs with water, bring to a boil, and place in the oven for 35 to 45 minutes, until the meat can be pulled off the bone easily.

3. Remove the bones from the chicken legs and place the meat back in the pot with the cooking liquid. Over medium heat, bring the pot to a boil. Continue to boil, cooking the liquid down until it has reduced to about ¾ cup.

4. Make the biscuits while the chicken is cooking. Combine the almond flour, butter, baking soda, eggs, and honey until they form a dough. Roll the dough into a ball or flat disc and place in the freezer for 15 minutes.

5. Place the dough between two parchment sheets and roll it out until it's about 1 inch thick. Cut into biscuit shapes; you can make the biscuits any size or shape you want, but be sure you end up with at least 4 to make the full recipe. If possible, chill the cut biscuits in the refrigerator for 10 to 15 minutes before baking; they will hold their shape and texture better.

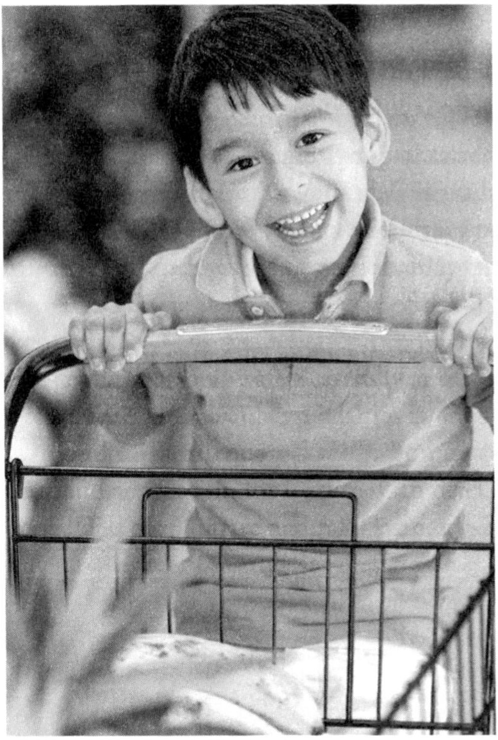

6. Bake the biscuits for 12 to 15 minutes, until golden brown. Serve the biscuits with the braised chicken and the reduced pan juices, or "gravy."

— *Travis H. Bettinson, Personal Chef, Seattle, Washington, www.junipfoods.com*

Chicken Lasagna

MAKES 8 SERVINGS

I created this recipe in hopes of giving loads of pleasure to those who thought taste was a thing of the past. Madeline, age 11, is not a red-sauce kinda girl, but this recipe passed the test. The more layers, the better; they give the lasagna better stability. And don't skimp on the cheese!

2 pounds ground chicken, turkey, or beef (or use a combination)
1 small yellow or white onion, finely chopped (optional)
3 cloves garlic, minced (or substitute ground garlic)
1½ cups dry curd cottage cheese
¼ cup freshly grated Parmesan cheese, divided
1 egg
8 leaves fresh basil, cut into chiffonade
1 (16-ounce) jar sugarless, SCD-friendly marinara sauce (I prefer Kirkland Signatures brand)
2 large zucchini, sliced lengthwise into strips about ¼ inch wide (remove the seeds if the zucchini is extra large)
2 cups SCD-legal hard cheese, mixed (such as Kerrygold Dubliner Cheddar with Monterey Jack)

1. Preheat the oven to 350°F.

2. Brown the meat in a large skillet over medium-high heat. Add the onion and garlic, stirring until soft, then drain off any extra fat. Add the jar of marinara and bring to a simmer. Turn off the heat.

3. In a separate bowl, combine the dry curd cottage cheese, half of the Parmesan cheese, the egg, and basil. Stir well and set aside.

4. In a 9-by-13-inch casserole dish, spread a thin layer of the prepared red sauce on the bottom, followed by a layer of sliced zucchini. Next, dot some dollops of the cottage cheese mixture over the zucchini and sprinkle a little of the hard cheese over that. Repeat with additional layers of sauce, zucchini, and hard cheese, building as many layers as you can. Finish with a nice layer of sauce and cheese.

5. Cover with foil (make it tight on the sides, but try to leave a dome of foil so the cheese doesn't stick to it). Pop the lasagna in the oven for 50 minutes. Remove the foil and sprinkle the remaining Parmesan on top; bake for another 10 minutes. Let the lasagna cool and settle for at least 10 minutes before serving.

— Stacey, SCD mom from Alabama

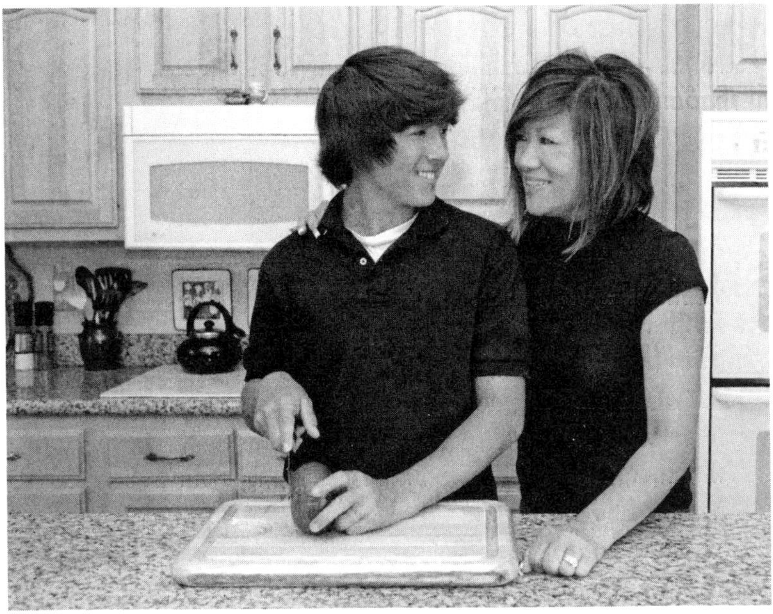

Zucchini "Fettuccine" Alfredo

Makes 3 servings

For those of you who are having white cheese sauce or béchamel withdrawals, I suggest you pay close attention. This recipe is sure to delight your taste buds and give those children of yours a true treat! Madeline, age 11, LOVED her fettuccine Alfredo before SCD. She didn't care if it involved gluten-free noodles or not—after all, it was the sauce that was the pièce de résistance.

Once I became proficient cooking in the SCD ways (and endured my fair share of failures!), this sauce came to be one night when I relied on intuition, familiar flavors, and the irresistible cashew to knock this one out of the park. My girl's response, "Are you serious? I can eat this? Thirds, please!"

3 medium zucchini
2 tablespoons extra-virgin olive oil
Salt and freshly ground pepper
1 cup cashews, soaked in water for at least 3 to 4 hours (can substitute macadamia nuts)
3 to 4 tablespoons ghee or butter
4 to 5 garlic cloves, minced
2 cups homemade chicken broth (recipe on page 136)
½ cup freshly grated Parmesan cheese
Pinch of nutmeg (optional)
1 sprig of fresh rosemary or thyme

1. Using either a mandolin or a good sharp knife, cut the zucchinis lengthwise into long, flat strips about ¼ inch wide. (You may want to discard the innermost, seedy strips, as they tend to fall apart when cooked.) Then cut the strips into "noodles" that resemble fettuccine or spaghetti.

2. Put the olive oil into a large sauté pan and set over medium-high heat. In one or two batches, stir-fry the zucchini noodles, turning them frequently until they're soft and pliable but not falling apart. Add salt and pepper to taste while the noodles are cooking. Set aside.

3. Drain the cashews well and set them aside.

4. In a saucepan, melt the ghee. Add the minced garlic and stir until it's gently brown. Add the broth and heat until steaming. Carefully pour the hot broth into a blender; add the cashews and blend until the mixture has thickened and no bits are noticeable. (I use a Vitamix and set it to high speed for a minute or two.)

5. Return the sauce to the saucepan and add the Parmesan cheese, plus the nutmeg if you're using it (no thank you for me!). You may vary the amount of cheese, depending on your desired consistency.

6. Toss the warm zucchini noodles with the Alfredo sauce and serve garnished with a sprig of rosemary or thyme.

— *Stacey, SCD mom from Alabama*

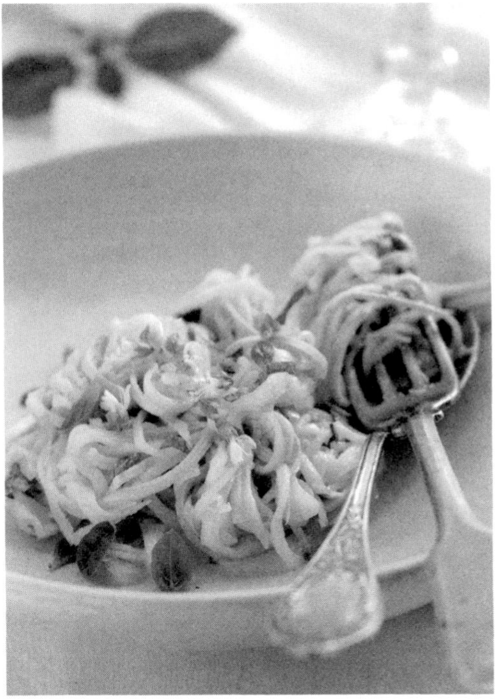

Fish Tacos

Makes about 6 tacos

This is a recipe I created when craving some good, healthy, SCD-friendly fish tacos. It helps so much to make a super-flavorful marinade for the fish and then to top the taco with an equally delicious, creamy, yogurt-cilantro sauce. Note that if your family prefers, this recipe works great using chicken or pork instead of the fish.

Sauce

2 cloves garlic
Freshly squeezed juice of ½ lime
½ cup homemade SCD yogurt
1 bunch fresh cilantro
2 green onions
1 roasted green bell pepper
Salt and freshly ground pepper

Marinade

1 tablespoon cumin powder
1 teaspoon paprika
1 handful fresh cilantro
2 whole garlic cloves, plus 2 minced cloves
Freshly squeezed juice from ½ lime
Salt and freshly ground pepper
¼ cup olive oil

1 pound boneless tilapia or other white fish
Cabbage, shredded
6 SCD taco shells (see the note below)

1. To make the sauce, use a blender or food processor to blend the garlic, lime juice, yogurt, cilantro, green onions, roasted green pepper, salt, and pepper. Once creamy, set aside.
2. To make the marinade, mix the cumin, paprika, cilantro, whole and minced garlic, lime juice, and a dash of salt and pepper in a small, shallow baking pan or pie plate. Add the olive oil and place the fish in the marinade, turning it until evenly coated.

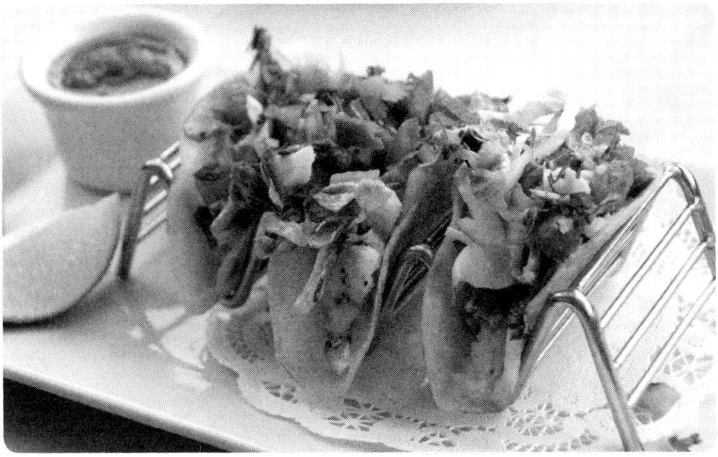

3. Heat the oven to 450°F. Cook the fish (still in the marinade) for 10 to 15 minutes, depending on the thickness of the fillets. When the fish is flaky and opaque all the way through, use two forks to separate it into small chunks. Set aside.

4. Heat several SCD tortillas (or use corn tortillas for family members who may prefer them). Add some shredded fish and shredded cabbage, top with a generous drizzle of sauce, and enjoy!

— Dr. Sara, Montana, an ER physician and SCD mom

Note: Your local supermarket may or may not carry ready-made, SCD-legal taco shells or tortillas. You can look online for them, or search for SCD-friendly recipes and make your own. Most use coconut flour, almond flour, cauliflower, or white beans as their base. Once you've found a recipe you like, it can be used to make taco shells, crepes, or even pizza dough.

Halibut with Mango Salsa

MAKES 2 SERVINGS

SALSA

2 large ripe mangoes, cubed
1 large tomato, cubed
¼ small red onion, finely minced
1 large clove garlic, finely minced
1 lime, juiced (1½ tablespoons)
¼ cup olive oil
Salt and freshly ground pepper
½ bunch fresh cilantro, chopped

8 ounces halibut fillet, cut into two pieces

1. To make the salsa, put all of the ingredients except the halibut into a large bowl; toss to combine. (This recipe makes more salsa that you will probably need for 2 servings, but it's so delicious and versatile that you'll enjoy using it in other ways.) Set the salsa aside.

2. Fill a pot with several inches of water (enough to submerge the halibut). Place over high heat. When it comes to a simmer, add the halibut, reduce the heat, and let it cook gently for 6 to 8 minutes, until cooked through.

3. Remove the halibut, drain on paper toweling, and serve with the mango salsa.

— *Travis H. Bettinson, Personal Chef, Seattle, Washington, www.junipfoods.com*

Braised Beef, Veggies, and Gravy

Makes 4 to 6 servings

I finally tried making gravy with pureed cooked veggies and drippings from the cooked meat, and the whole family absolutely loved it—even the hubby! I'm glad I finally tried the gravy prior to Thanksgiving—it's fantastic!

1½ cups water (or use homemade meat broth or vegetable stock)
3 cups small cauliflower florets
1 to 3 sprigs fresh rosemary, each about 6 inches long
1 to 3 sprigs fresh sage
1½ to 2 pounds stewing beef
Salt and freshly ground pepper
2 to 3 cups of other vegetables to cook with the meat (carrots and onions are always good)

1. Pour the water into a Crock-Pot or a slow cooker and add the cauliflower, rosemary, and sage. Next, season the beef with salt and pepper; add other veggies you want to cook with the meat. Following the guidelines provided by the Crock-Pot or slow cooker manufacturer, cook for as long as is advised for the cut of meat you've chosen—typically about 8 hours on low.

2. Transfer the meat to a serving dish and cover to keep it warm. Using a slotted spoon, transfer the cooked vegetables into a bowl to cool. Remove and discard the spent herbs.

3. Put the vegetables and all of the liquid into a blender. Cover with the lid, but first remove the inner part of the lid so the steam can vent freely. (Alternatively, keep the vegetables in the pot and puree using an immersion blender.) Blend until very smooth; season with more salt and pepper to taste. Pour the gravy into a serving dish, divide the meat between warmed plates, and enjoy!

— Barbara, SCD mom from Washington

Pecan-Crusted Orange Roughy

Makes 4 servings

This is a family favorite! If you can't find orange roughy, cod, red snapper, or halibut will work great as substitutes.

1⁄3 cup almond flour (we prefer the Honeyville brand)
1⁄8 to 1⁄4 cup finely chopped pecans
1 teaspoon chopped parsley
1⁄2 teaspoon paprika
1⁄4 teaspoon SCD-legal garlic salt
Dash regular salt
1 egg
2 tablespoons melted butter
4 fillets orange roughy

1. Preheat the oven to 350°F. Grease a glass baking dish or a baking sheet with butter or olive oil and set aside.

2. In a shallow bowl, mix the flour, pecans, parsley, paprika, garlic salt, and regular salt until well combined. Whisk the egg and melted butter in a separate bowl.

3. Dip each orange roughy fillet into the egg mixture, then into the flour mixture. Put into the baking dish. Bake for 20 to 30 minutes, or until crisp and golden brown.

— Stephanie, SCD mom from Indiana

Breaded Chicken Strips

Makes 3 to 4 servings

Our son was diagnosed with Crohn's disease at age 12. He has been on the SCD for almost three years, and he is doing very well. I remind myself often that I'm cooking from scratch—just like my grandma used to! Planning meals ahead is a great help. We are so thankful for this diet, which allows him to be just like any normal teenager!

Olive oil or butter, for greasing the pan
1½ cups almond flour
¾ teaspoon salt
¼ teaspoon freshly ground pepper
¼ teaspoon SCD-legal garlic salt (optional)
¼ teaspoon SCD-legal onion salt (optional)
1 egg, well beaten
1 pound chicken tenders (or use breasts sliced into strips)

1. Heat the oven to 350°F. Lightly grease the bottom of a glass dish or baking sheet with olive oil or butter.

2. In a shallow bowl, mix the flour, salt, pepper, garlic salt, and onion salt until well combined. Put the beaten egg into a small bowl.

3. Dip the chicken pieces into the egg, then roll them in the flour mixture, coating all sides. Place the chicken into the baking dish and bake for 30 to 45 minutes, or until crisp and golden brown. Honey, SCD-legal barbecue sauce, or mustard make great dipping sauces.

— Stephanie, SCD mom from Indiana

Sloppy Joe Mix

Makes 4 servings

All kids like Sloppy Joes, and this version is very tasty and satisfying. You can use it as an entrée (I like to serve it over cooked spaghetti squash or zucchini, or alongside any steamed or roasted veggie), or add several spoonfuls to scrambled eggs or omelets.

1 tablespoon olive oil
1 medium onion, finely chopped
1 pound good-quality ground beef
2 cloves garlic
½ teaspoon dried thyme, or 2 teaspoons chopped fresh thyme leaves
½ teaspoon dried sage, or 1 teaspoon chopped fresh sage leaves
1 teaspoon paprika
Pinch of cayenne pepper
½ cup SCD-legal ketchup, or 3 medium tomatoes cooked with salt and your choice of herbs
Salt and freshly ground pepper

1. Heat a large sauté pan over medium heat with the olive oil. Add the onion and cook, stirring occasionally until soft and golden brown. Add the ground beef and cook, stirring, until brown.

2. Add the garlic, thyme, sage, paprika, and cayenne. Stir to combine. Add the ketchup or cooked tomatoes. Season to taste with salt, pepper, and more cayenne, if desired. Simmer for about 30 minutes, or until most of the liquid has evaporated.

— *Tanya, SCD mom from Washington*

Sweet and Sour Chicken

Makes 4 servings

1 medium orange, cut into chunks
2 cups fresh pineapple chunks
3 tablespoons honey
2 tablespoons apple cider vinegar
2 tablespoons sesame oil
1 pound boneless, skinless chicken breasts, cut into bite-size pieces
Salt and freshly ground pepper
1 large green bell pepper, diced
1 large red bell pepper, diced
1 small onion, diced
3 cloves garlic, chopped
2 tablespoons ginger, grated

1. Using a blender, puree the orange, pineapple, honey, and vinegar until smooth. Balance the flavor to your preference by adding more honey or vinegar.

2. Place a sauté pan over medium-high heat for 2 to 3 minutes; add the sesame oil to coat the bottom of the pan. Add the chicken, season it with salt and pepper, and sauté for 3 to 4 minutes, turning occasionally, until golden brown.

3. Remove the chicken from the pan and add the bell peppers, onion, garlic, and ginger. Sauté for 3 to 4 minutes until the veggies are slightly softened and aromatic.

4. Put the chicken back into the pan, then add the orange-pineapple puree. Bring to a simmer and cook for 5 minutes, allowing the flavors to combine.

— *Travis H. Bettinson, Personal Chef, Seattle, Washington, www.junipfoods.com*

Baked "Spaghetti" with Two Cheeses

MAKES 6 TO 8 SERVINGS

If you haven't tried spaghetti squash, you're in for a treat! This light yellow, watermelon-shaped squash (most readily available in late fall and early winter) has a surprise to offer. When cooked and scraped from its rind, it falls out in perfect long strands that look a lot like real spaghetti noodles. Its rather bland-tasting flesh makes it a great foil for all kinds of sauces and preparations. Be sure your kids are standing by when you magically create noodles from a vegetable!

1 spaghetti squash (about 4 pounds—see the note below)
1 pound lean ground beef
1 (24-ounce) jar SCD-legal spaghetti sauce
2 cups shredded cheddar cheese (see the note below)
1 cup freshly grated Parmesan cheese (see the note below)

1. Heat the oven to 375°F.

2. Bake the spaghetti squash by cutting it in half lengthwise and placing it flesh side down in a baking dish. Bake for about 45 minutes, or until tender. (You can also cook it in a microwave. Poke the rind several times with a fork, and place it in a microwave-safe dish. Cook on high power for about 10 minutes, or until tender.) When the squash is cooked, scoop out the seeds and strings and discard. Using a fork, scrape the flesh of the squash into a large bowl; it should resemble spaghetti noodles. If it is watery, place it in a colander to drain.

3. While the squash is baking, brown the ground beef in a large saucepan over medium heat, draining any excess fat. Pour in the spaghetti sauce and simmer for about 10 minutes, or until the sauce has thickened slightly.

4. Lower the oven temperature to 350°F.

5. To assemble, lay the squash "noodles" in the bottom of a 9-by-13-inch baking dish (you probably won't need all of the squash; refrigerate any extra for another use). Add the cheddar cheese in an even layer. Ladle the meat sauce over the cheese and top with the Parmesan (you can add more cheddar on top if you'd like).

6. Bake at 350°F for about 30 minutes. You can't really overbake this—my family likes it when the cheese has browned and the dish is bubbling.

— Stephanie, SCD mom from Indiana

Notes: Spaghetti squashes often run on the large size, with an average weight of 4 to 8 pounds. Ask your produce person to cut one in half for you, or offer to share half with a friend. Or cook the entire squash and try it a couple of different ways.

We have a "salad shooter" kitchen tool that we use to shred or grate bars of aged cheeses. We freeze the shredded or grated cheese in containers to have on hand as needed.

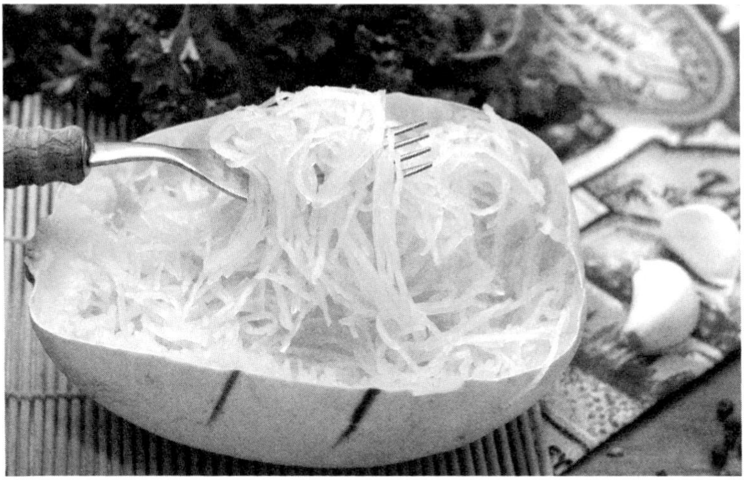

Cauliflower Pizza Crust MAKES 1 MEDIUM PIZZA CRUST

Have fun with the wonderful flavors of fresh herbs here! Thyme, oregano, rosemary, basil, or parsley are all wonderful, alone or in combination.

1 medium head cauliflower
1 large egg
½ cup freshly grated Parmesan or shredded mozzarella cheese, loosely packed
2 teaspoons fresh herbs, or 1 teaspoon dried herbs
¼ teaspoon salt
¼ teaspoon freshly ground pepper
Assorted SCD-legal pizza toppings of your choice

1. Preheat the oven to 375°F. Line a round pizza pan with parchment paper (a heavy baking sheet will also work fine). Cut a large square of cheesecloth, double or triple it, and set it over a medium bowl.

2. Rinse the cauliflower, remove the outer leaves, and cut it into florets. Put the florets into a food processor and whirl until they have the texture of rice (some coarser chunks are fine). Spread the cauliflower onto the parchment-lined baking sheet and bake for 15 minutes. Let it sit until it's cool enough to handle.

3. Transfer the cooked cauliflower to the cheesecloth-lined bowl, then squeeze the liquid out of it. Be patient and do this a few times until barely any liquid comes out. Muscle work!

4. Increase the oven temperature to 450°F.

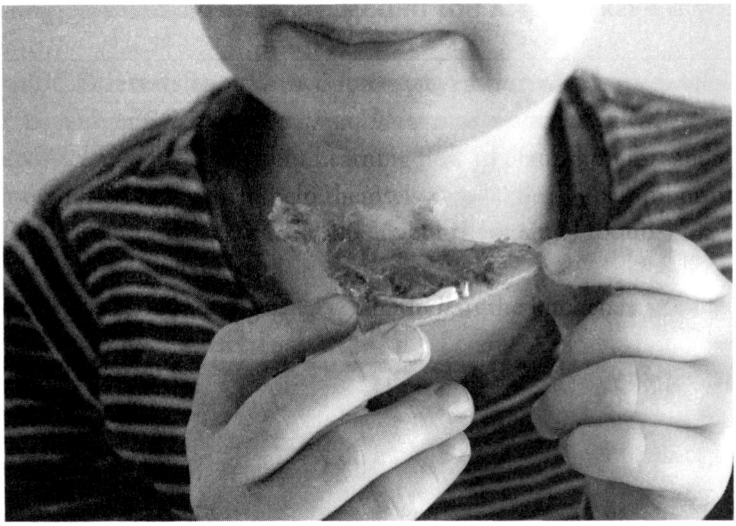

5. Transfer the cauliflower to a mixing bowl along with the egg, cheese, herbs, salt, and pepper; mix to combine, then pour it onto the baking sheet. Flatten and shape the mixture until it resembles a thin pizza crust. Bake for 15 to 20 minutes. Note that the crust will get dark golden brown on the edges before it has browned in the center. Be patient and allow it get there, even if you are getting nervous about burning the outside. It will be fine.

6. Add your favorite toppings and bake again until they are hot and the cheese is melted and golden brown.

— *Olena, www.ifoodreal.com*

Tarte Flambé from Alsace

Makes 4 servings (One 12-inch tart)

Tarte flambé is, in essence, a pizza with white sauce and a very thin, crisp crust. This is a version that roughly follows the classic combination of smoky bacon, onion, herbs, and soft, fresh cheese—but you can and should improvise on the toppings, using whatever pizza-like ingredients you and your family love.

Topping

Several slices bacon or ham
¼ cup finely chopped onion
1 tablespoon chopped fresh chives or chopped fresh thyme (optional)

Dough

1 egg white
½ cup almond flour, plus more as needed to make a workable dough
1 tablespoon olive oil

1 cup SCD yogurt

1. Fry the bacon or ham in a pan until crisp; add the onion, and cook briefly. (You can also add other SCD-legal topping ingredients of your choice to this mixture.) Set aside.

2. Place a rack in the lower third of the oven; preheat to 375°F.

3. Mix the dough ingredients thoroughly in a small bowl, then roll the dough between two layers of parchment paper until very thin (add more flour as necessary to reduce sticking). Remove the upper paper, then slide the lower paper, along with the crust, into the oven. Bake for 5 to 7 minutes, checking regularly, until the crust is light golden brown. If it seems to be baking too fast, lower the temperature.

4. Remove from the oven and distribute the toppings evenly over the crust. Drizzle with yogurt (if it is too thick to drizzle, thin it with a little warm water). Return the tarte to the oven and bake for 5 minutes more, or until the toppings are hot. Serve immediately.

— Morana, SCD mom from Switzerland

Tomato, Cauliflower, and Cheese Frittata

Makes 2 servings

4 eggs
2 plum tomatoes, chopped
½ small white onion, diced
3 cloves garlic, minced
½ small head cauliflower, finely chopped
⅓ cup olive oil
1 tablespoon salt
1 tablespoon freshly ground pepper

1. Preheat the oven to 350°F.

2. Whisk the eggs in a large bowl, then add the tomatoes.

3. Put the onion, garlic, cauliflower, oil, salt, and pepper into a large, oven-safe sauté pan (no plastic handles, please!). Place the pan over low to medium-low heat (you don't want to brown the ingredients) and cook the mixture for 7 to 10 minutes, stirring, until everything is soft and hot.

4. Pour the vegetables into the egg-tomato mixture, and stir to combine (this will partially cook the eggs).

5. Pour the mixture back into the sauté pan. Using a rubber spatula, move the mixture around as if scrambling eggs until the eggs are mostly set. Place the pan in the oven for 5 minutes and bake until all of the ingredients have set. Cool slightly, cut, and serve.

— Travis H. Bettinson, Personal Chef, Seattle, Washington, www.junipfoods.com

Tuna Patties

MAKES FOUR (3-INCH) PATTIES

2 (5-ounce) cans SCD-legal tuna in water only, drained
2 tablespoons finely chopped celery
2 teaspoons finely chopped onion
1 egg
Salt and freshly ground pepper
1 tablespoon butter

1. In a medium bowl, mix the tuna, celery, onion, and egg. Season to taste with salt and pepper.

2. Heat the butter in a small skillet over medium heat. Shape portions of the tuna mixture as you would hamburgers. Place the patties in the skillet. Gently flip the patties when browned on one side and cook the other side. They are done when browned on both sides.

— *Stephanie, SCD mom from Indiana*

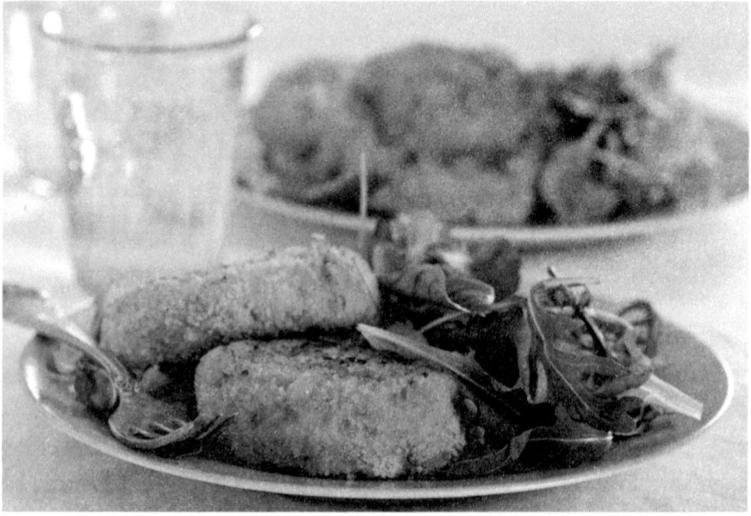

Baked Tuna with Tomato, Basil, and Olives

Makes 4 servings

1 pound (about 4 medium) tomatoes, chopped
2 tablespoons capers
½ cup pitted Kalamata olives, chopped
1 bunch fresh basil
Salt and freshly ground pepper
3 tablespoons extra-virgin olive oil
4 (1-inch thick) albacore tuna steaks (about 2 pounds)

1. Preheat the oven to 350°F.

2. Toss the tomatoes, capers, olives, basil, salt, and pepper in a bowl.

3. Pour the olive oil into a 9-by-13-inch baking dish and spread evenly. Lay the pieces of tuna in the pan, turning them to coat evenly with oil. Distribute the tomato mixture on top of the tuna. Bake for about 25 minutes, or until the fish is baked through and the vegetables have softened and begun to release their juices.

— *Travis H. Bettinson, Personal Chef, Seattle, Washington, www.junipfoods.com*

Braised Ground Turkey with Almonds

MAKES 4 SERVINGS

This is a simple way to cook ground turkey so that it's extra tasty and moist. A simple side dish of steamed lentils or a bounteous spinach salad would be great accompaniments.

3 tablespoons olive oil
1 pound ground turkey
1 large onion, chopped
3 cloves garlic, chopped
2 Roma tomatoes, diced
2 tablespoons almonds, toasted and chopped
1 bay leaf
Salt and freshly ground pepper

1. Heat a large saucepot over medium-high heat for 2 to 3 minutes. Add the olive oil. Crumble the turkey into the pan and sear until it's brown on one side.

2. Remove the turkey from the pot. Add the onion, garlic, tomatoes, almonds, and bay leaf; sauté for 2 to 3 minutes, until the vegetables soften. Season to taste with salt and pepper.

3. Add the turkey back to the pot along with enough water to barely cover the meat. Bring to a simmer. Continue simmering for about 30 minutes, or until the liquid has mostly evaporated and the flavors have combined.

— Travis H. Bettinson, Personal Chef, Seattle, Washington, www.junipfoods.com

Zucchini Bread

MAKES ONE (5-BY-7-INCH) LOAF CAKE

2 large eggs
½ cup honey
¼ cup (½ stick) butter, melted and cooled
¼ teaspoon freshly grated ginger
¼ teaspoon freshly grated nutmeg
2 cups almond flour
½ teaspoon baking soda
1½ cups grated zucchini

1. Preheat the oven to 350°F. Grease a 5-by-7-inch loaf pan generously with butter.

2. Using a stand mixer fitted with the paddle attachment or a hand-held electric mixer, blend the eggs with the honey until smooth. Add the butter, ginger, and nutmeg; mix until smooth. Add the almond flour and the baking soda, and mix until just incorporated. Add the zucchini and use a spoon to gently blend it into the batter.

3. Pour the batter into the baking pan and bake for about 60 minutes, or until a toothpick inserted into the center comes out clean.

— Stephanie, SCD mom from Indiana

Almond Cake

MAKES ONE (5-BY-7-INCH) LOAF CAKE

This batter can be used to make cupcakes as well. Bake them at 300°F for 15 to 20 minutes.

1 cup (8 ounces) SCD-legal almond butter, homemade or purchased
6 tablespoons (¾ stick) butter, at room temperature
2 large eggs
2 egg yolks
⅓ cup honey
2 tablespoons almond flour

1. Preheat the oven to 300°F. Generously grease a 5-by-7-inch loaf pan and set aside.

2. Make a double boiler to melt the almond butter and regular butter: First, put both into a medium metal bowl. Put an inch or so of water into a slightly larger pot and bring it to a simmer. Set the bowl over the bigger pot. As the butter melts, whisk it with the almond butter until a smooth paste forms. Remove the bowl from the pot and set it aside to cool to room temperature.

3. Using a stand mixer fitted with the whisk attachment (or using a hand-held mixer), whisk the eggs, the extra egg yolks, and the honey. Whip on high for 2 to 3 minutes, until the mixture has frothed up to about 1½ times its original volume.

4. Put the almond mixture—it should be just slightly warm or at room temperature—into a large, wide bowl. Use a rubber spatula to scrape about a quarter of the egg mixture into the bowl. Stir gently to combine—at this point you don't have to be too careful, since your goal is to lighten the heavy almond and butter paste so that the next steps are easier.

5. Now begin the folding process: Put half of the remaining egg mixture into the bowl and cut through the two mixtures with the edge of the

spatula. Turn your wrist as you pull the spatula through the center of the bowl, sweeping the spatula through, over, and back under the egg mixture. With the other hand, turn the bowl as you make this motion. Your goal is to keep as much air in the batter as possible while blending the two mixtures. Repeat with the last of the egg mixture.

6. When the almond paste and eggs are *mostly* blended (they don't have to be completely uniform, since you'll be doing more folding), sprinkle the almond flour over the top of the mixture. Use the same gentle folding motions to incorporate the almond flour.

7. Pour the batter into the pan and place it in the oven. Bake for about 40 minutes, or until a toothpick inserted into the center comes out clean.

8. Because there is a lot of egg in this cake, you should not leave it at room temperature. Store it, well wrapped, in the refrigerator.

— *Travis H. Bettinson, Personal Chef, Seattle, Washington, www.junipfoods.com*

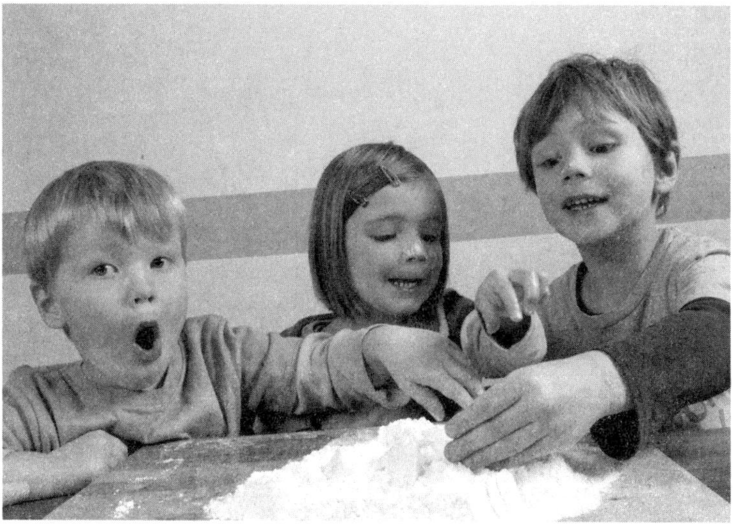

Caramel-Pear Upside-Down Cake

MAKES ONE (9- TO 10-INCH) ROUND CAKE

Note from Morana: We are very grateful that we came across this diet soon after our son was diagnosed with Crohn's disease. In particular, we are very grateful for the support from the SCD families Facebook group—it helps us feel less isolated here far away where we do not know anybody else doing this diet.

6 ounces (1½ sticks) butter, divided
½ cup honey
2 to 3 ripe pears (other fruit, such as apples, plums, or peaches may be used instead)
Cinnamon (optional)
2 eggs
5 ounces (1¼ cups) almond flour
½ teaspoon baking soda
Pinch of salt

1. Place a rack in the lower third of the oven; preheat the oven to 350°F.

2. Melt 2 ounces (½ stick) of the butter in a pan and add ¼ cup of the honey. Stir to combine, then pour into the cake pan and distribute evenly.

3. Peel and thinly slice the pears; sprinkle them with cinnamon if you like.

4. To make the batter, melt the remaining 4 ounces (1 stick) of butter; set it aside to cool. Using an electric mixer (or a large bowl and spoon), blend the butter with the remaining ¼ cup of honey, eggs, almond flour, baking soda, and salt until smooth.

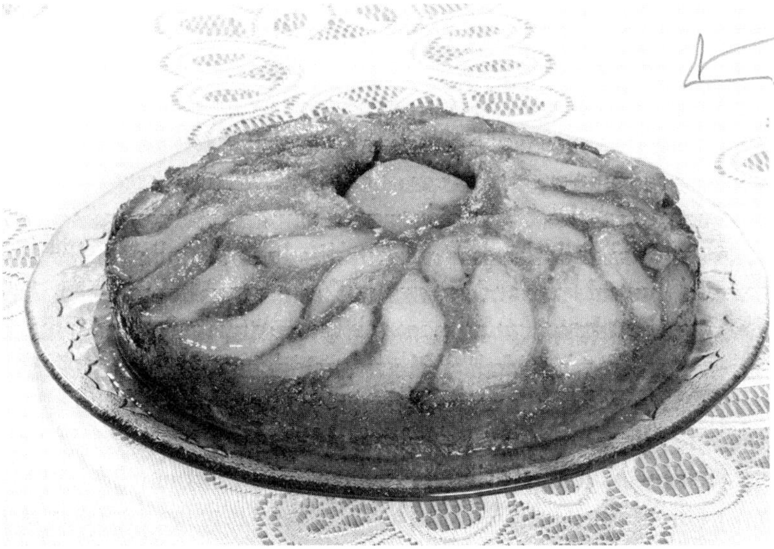

5. Arrange the pear slices in overlapping circles in the pan. Slowly pour the batter over them, being careful not to displace the slices. Bake for about 25 minutes, or until golden brown. After the cake has cooled a little bit, flip it from the pan onto a cake platter so that the caramelized pears are on the top. (Be sure to do this while the cake is still warm, as the caramel will set up as it cools, making it impossible to remove from the pan!)

— Morana, SCD mom from Switzerland

Swiss Meringue Buttercream Icing

Makes 4 cups

Have patience when making this icing. When the butter is being mixed in, you will look at the icing dozens of times, thinking, "I messed up and it has broken." THAT IS NOT TRUE. The icing will appear runny and possibly curdled until it finally (sometimes after 40 minutes of slow mixing) turns into a smooth icing. Patience is key.

5 egg whites
1 cup mild honey
1 pound (4 sticks) butter, cubed and at room temperature

1. Put the egg whites and honey in a medium stainless steel bowl; whisk to combine. Place the bowl over a slightly larger pot that contains simmering water. Whisk slowly but continuously for 5 minutes, until the mixture is hot. If you see the egg whites begin to set up, immediately remove the bowl from the heat, continuing to whisk to stop the cooking—then place the bowl back over the pot to complete the 5 minutes of cooking.

2. Pour the mixture into a stand mixer fitted with the whisk attachment. Using the highest speed, whisk for 4 to 5 minutes. The mixture will turn into a Swiss meringue, meaning that the egg whites will fluff up and form stiff peaks. Note that it's better to have very stiff peaks than ones that are softer, so if you have to whisk the egg white mixture for longer, it's okay.

3. Replace the whisk attachment with the paddle. Turn the mixer to low speed (#2) and add the butter little by little (adding it too fast will break the icing and it will not set properly). This should take 2 to 3 minutes. When all of the butter has been added, walk away for 25 to 30 minutes, letting the mixer continue to mix the butter and egg whites. If the icing has not come together in this time (meaning that it will look slightly runny and curdled), just walk away and come back every 10 minutes until it looks and feels like a typical cake icing.

4. Remove the icing from the bowl and spread onto anything you wish. Store in the refrigerator for up to 2 weeks.

— Travis H. Bettinson, Personal Chef, Seattle, Washington, www.junipfoods.com

How to Know If the SCD Is Working for You

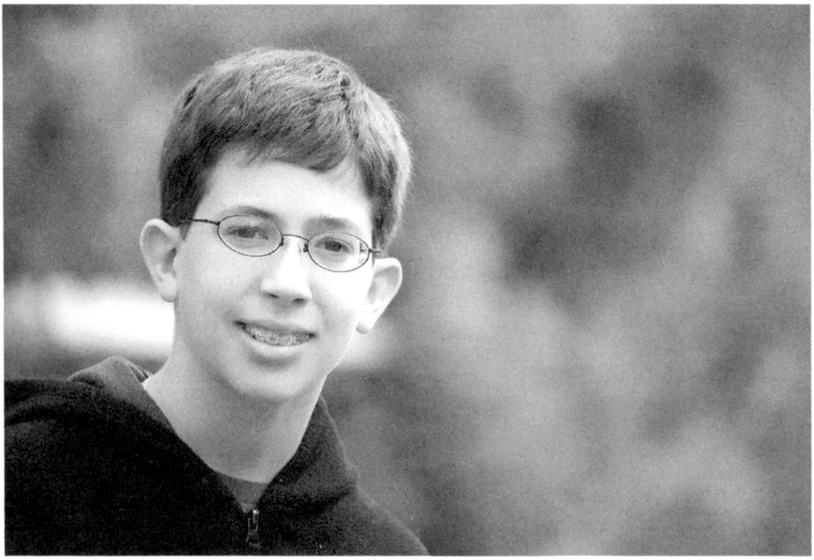

Knowing Your Child's Disease:
How to Know If Your Child's Treatment is Working

Which patients are the most successful at managing IBD? Which are more likely to stay in remission?

Individuals and families who make it a point to learn as much as they can about the disease are the ones who best understand what's happening. And because of their efforts, they are the ones who are most likely to stay in remission.

While many reasons exist as to why one person might do better than another, understanding what's happening and learning as much as you can is a necessary step in the right direction. And it's a first step toward managing IBD problems.

Why?

The healthcare providers you see are experts in their fields, concerned about your care, treatment, and outcome. However, their decisions are mostly based on what you tell them. You should want to be the perfect partner with your healthcare providers. For that, you have to make sure you're accurate and honest in what you tell them. In fact you, your healthcare providers, *and* your child have got to be a team to ensure the very best possible outcomes.

So, in that light, it is essential that you and your child understand IBD and everything about it. Everybody's IBD "presents" (how it appears in your child) differently. Here are some of the questions you should be thinking about to discuss with your doctor:

What were your child's first symptoms?

How did you first recognize that there was a problem? Knowing this helps you predict what the warning signs will be when your child has flares (relapses) or increased symptoms.

You may be wondering what the usual symptoms are. Generally they include the following:

- Diarrhea
- Abdominal pain
- Fevers

- Oral ulcerations
- Joint pains
- Rashes

Of course, you should note any other symptoms you've noticed and be sure to mention them to your doctor. The severity of these symptoms may vary. Your job is to "track" their severity to determine how well your child (or you, if you are the patient) is doing.

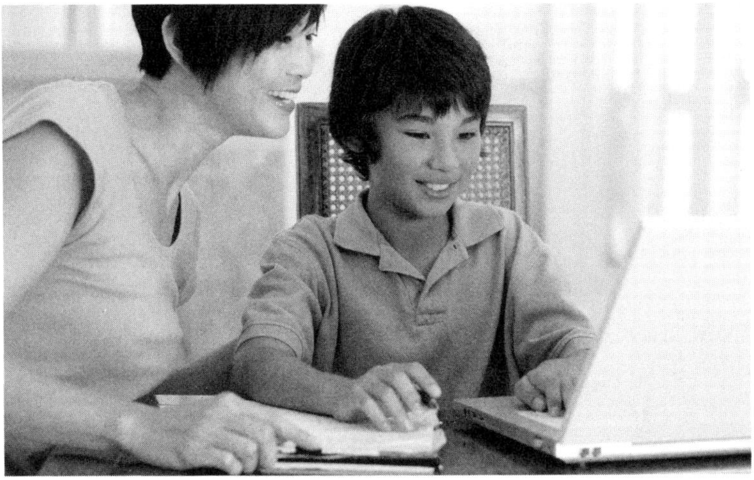

What do we mean by "tracking?"

At Children's, children with Crohn's disease and ulcerative colitis are tracked—that is, monitored for disease activity. Tracking means keeping a written account of the patient's symptoms over time. For example, if the main symptom is bloody diarrhea, make a note of each episode of diarrhea, its consistency, how much blood it contains, and anything else that seems important.

Here is an example:

> **Monday, June 17**
> *5 bowel movements, mostly watery with blood in 3 of them.*
> *No stomach pain.*

This will help your child's healthcare team assess the severity of the flare and what treatment is indicated. The level of flare activity is defined by a specific score. I will describe these scores in the next few pages. These scores give us a solid idea as to how well a patient is doing, how effective a particular therapy is, or if other therapy should be considered.

Tracking is not instinctive, but it is essential. Learning how to properly do it helps you explain the degree of illness in a way that is understandable to your child, yourself, and your healthcare provider. Tracking how an individual is doing helps provide the best care for your child by giving objective information that can be followed over time. While tracking is important, it's also fairly simple to learn. I promise that you, as a parent or caregiver, will have very little problem learning how to do it.

Here are my suggestions:

Relax.
(Actually, that may be the hardest part! But it's a very important part.)

Don't over-analyze!
(That is, worry, worry, worry!)

As a parent myself, this is easier said than done! But it's important not to get hung up on the small details and lose sight of the big picture. Don't question your child every minute about how they feel. That is, don't worry, worry, worry and don't ask, ask, ask. Checking in weekly or even monthly will work just fine for establishing how things are going for your child. Besides, as a parent or caregiver, you will recognize plenty of nonverbal cues in your child that gives clues as to how they feel (energy level, fatigue, hurting tummy, etc.).

Perspective is very important. If we overreact, there's a chance we might overtreat; if we underreact we might undertreat. Remember, you're part of a team. Stand back and take a deep breath. Discuss things with your healthcare provider and with other parents. This can help give you a sense of the best way to handle things.

Give yourself time. It won't be long until *you* will be the expert helping other parents who are just beginning the process of managing their child's disease.

PCDAI and PUCAI scores

Now, about those scores.

The formal name of the score for pediatric Crohn's disease is the Pediatric Crohn's Disease Activity Index, or PCDAI. (Adult patients have different but similar scores.) Depending on how many symptoms are present and their severity, the PCDAI lets your child's doctor know if your child is likely in remission (our goal!), having mild to moderate disease activity, or experiencing severe disease activity.

What determines these scores?

- Abdominal pain
- Stools per day
- Overall patient well-being

- Laboratory exams, including—
    - Hematocrit
    - Sedimentation rate
    - Albumin

- Physical exams, including—
    - Weight
    - Height
    - Abdominal tenderness
    - Perirectal exam
    - Other intestinal manifestations
    - Fever greater than 101.3°F (38.5°C) for 3 days over the previous week
    - Oral ulcerations
    - Definitive arthritis
    - Uveitis
    - Erythema nodosum (an IBD-associated rash)
    - Pyoderma gangrenosum (an IBD-associated rash)

Which PCDAI version should you be using?

While the PCDAI is helpful for physicians, it's more difficult to do at home because it relies on laboratory studies. In that case, and when laboratory studies cannot be done, the shortened PCDAI is effective. This primarily uses the symptoms of Crohn's (see the list above) to determine the severity of disease. While this may sound obvious to do—that is, follow the symptoms—oftentimes during the busy juggling of life, we and our children forget to track these symptoms. This can make it difficult to determine if somebody is doing better or worse or having no change at all.

The PUCAI

Children with ulcerative colitis, on the other hand, use a different scoring system—the Pediatric Ulcerative Colitis Activity Index (PUCAI). Its score is based on the assessment of the following symptoms:

- Abdominal pain
- Rectal bleeding
- Stool consistency
- Number of stools in a 24-hour period
- Nocturnal stools that awaken the patient
- The child's activity level

Similar to the PCDAI, depending on how many symptoms are present and their severity, the PUCAI lets your child's doctor know if your child is likely in remission (again our goal), having mild to moderate disease activity, or experiencing severe disease activity.

Laboratory testing

Another tool that is used to assess how well a person with IBD is doing is laboratory testing. For many patients, laboratory studies can show evidence of inflammation, anemia, and other signs of disease activity, although it is important to note that some people with IBD can have active disease with normal laboratory studies. Oftentimes you can find out if your child's laboratory studies indicate disease activity by seeing if lab abnormalities were present at their initial diagnosis. If they were, you'll then be reassured that normal labs are indicating that the disease is in check.

What laboratory tests are done?

1. **The complete blood count (CBC)**
   The CBC is an overall test for your blood, including —

- **Hemoglobin and hematocrit:** This measures the amount of red blood cells in the blood. Red blood cells help move oxygen through the body. The result of low red blood cell counts (i.e., anemia) includes fatigue, exhaustion, and decreased energy. More importantly, severe anemia can be life-threatening.

- **White blood count:** White blood cells help fight infection.

- **Platelets:** These are important for clotting blood.

In IBD, what do continuous abnormally low red-blood-cell counts indicate?

- Poor absorption of iron
- Bleeding in the GI tract
- Inflammation (as an indirect result)

… all of which may indicate active disease.

2. **Albumin levels**
   Albumin is a protein in the blood serum. Its purpose is to transport other molecules throughout the body. During active disease, decreased serum albumin is present in the blood because of losses in the gastrointestinal tract and decreased production in the liver. Once again, low levels indicate active disease.

3. **Erythrocyte sedimentation rate (ESR) and C-reactive protein (CRP)**
   These measure inflammation in the body.

   - **ESR:** This is a measure of inflammation within the body. The inflamed body makes many different types of proteins called "acute phase reactants." During this test, red blood cells (erythrocytes) fall into a small tube. If many acute phase reactants (i.e., inflammatory proteins) are present in the blood, it takes more time for red blood cells to fall to the bottom of the tube, and therefore we know your ESR is elevated. If red blood cells fall at a normal rate, the ESR is normal.

- **CRP:** This is a direct measure of inflammation in the body. CRP is a specific acute-phase reactant and protein produced by the liver in response to infection or other inflammatory states.

The difficulty with both the ESR and CRP is that they are not specific for inflammatory bowel disease and can be elevated by other inflammatory states such as colds, flu, and other infections.

4. **Stool calprotectin**
   Unlike ESR and CRP, stool calprotectin is a biochemical test specifically for intestinal inflammation. With inflammation in the bowels comes an increase in white blood cells in the intestines. Certain types of white blood cells make calprotectin; therefore, the stool calprotectin indirectly measures the amount of white blood cells and thus inflammation in the bowels. A handy aspect of stool calprotectin is that it tells you if the inflammation is directly in the bowels. This differs from ESR and CRP, which can be elevated if other inflammatory processes are going on outside of the bowels, such as a cold. However, the stool calprotectin levels do not differentiate between some gastrointestinal infections and inflammatory bowel disease.

Why should you know all of this?

The more you know and understand, the more comfortable you will be in asking questions. The more questions you ask, the more discussions you'll have, and thereby the more you, your child, and your healthcare provider are a team. With this team approach to healthcare, not only do you get better understanding of IBD, you get better outcomes. And, in the end, that is what we all want.

Alternatives to SCD

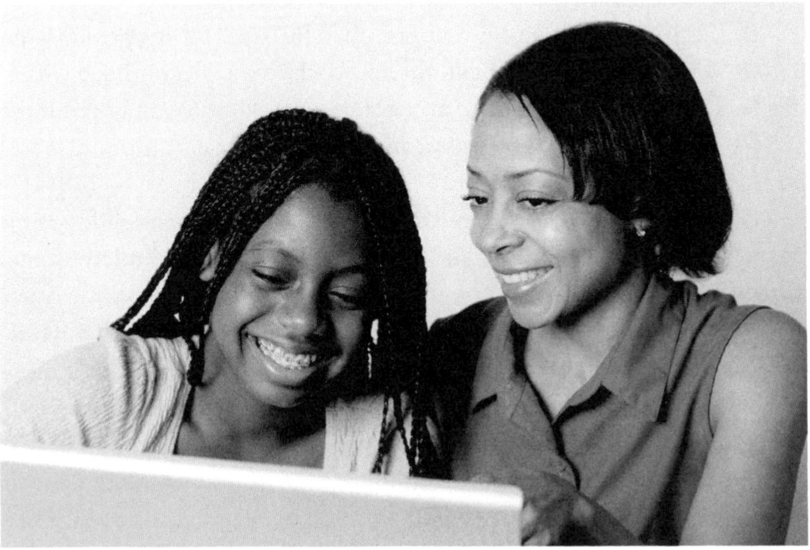

What If the SCD Doesn't Work?

Alternatives to SCD

What if you want to do the specific carbohydrate diet, but can't? Is it all or nothing? The answer is yes and no. We know that diet has a major impact on disease, and that the SCD works for patients with inflammatory bowel disease. And we are still learning about many specific aspects of the SCD and which ones are the most important. But we still don't know many things about the interaction of nutrition, diet, and disease.

But, if you are able and it is appropriate for you and your child to go on the SCD, I would recommend the approach to the diet outlined within this book. For some, going on it may not be a good option. But even if the SCD is not feasible and you are treating IBD with medication, diet still plays an important role.

Eating a healthy diet is important! Whether you or your child are on the SCD or not, what is eaten profoundly impacts the fecal microbiome. Two sides play a role in IBD—one is the immune system, and the other is the microbiome, to which the immune system is reacting. By avoiding foods that may harm your fecal microbiome and instead eating those that improve its biodiversity and health, you are likely to improve your disease. While this topic requires much more medical research, I feel that both avoiding highly processed foods—which usually come in cans or packages—and eating a more healthy, organic whole-foods diet result in a healthier microbiome, and therefore a healthier you.

Improving diets

My recommendations for improving diets are simple:

1. **Remove as many processed foods from your diet as possible,** especially junk food such as chips, soda pop, candies, cakes, and multi-ingredient packaged and processed foods. As my wife likes to say, if more than three ingredients are listed on the packaging, avoid it! Although the processed foods we eat can be tasty, they often contain items that we would not consider food.

   Take, for instance, Subway sandwiches. Recently, the company had issues with azodicarbonamide, a chemical that is used to bleach flour. It also happens to be a foaming agent in the plastics and rubber industry and thus is a key component of yoga mats. This additive is completely legal in the United States and is used in many food items, including the bread in Subway sandwiches. As with many human-made chemicals in our foods that we as general consumers just don't know much about, this additive would have continued to be present in Subway sandwiches had it not been for a large national public outcry, which pressured the company to remove it in early 2014.

Unfortunately, many other food additives exist whose effects on our bodies are not known, and because they may not be as mentally repulsive as the azodicarbonamide-and-yoga-mat connection or because consumers are not properly informed, they stay in our foods. In 1997 the Food and Drug Administration (FDA) succumbed to pressure from the food industry and politicians by creating a back door for food additives to come onto the market.[3] While some of these additives may be fine for human consumption, we don't always know if they really are, because rigorous safety testing is often not required to see if they are truly safe, especially over the long term. And these food additives are frequently present in our processed foods and drinks.

2. **Avoid eating out.** This brings us back to the reason in Item 1. Once again, we don't always know what we are eating when we consume mass-made foods. They look and smell delicious and probably taste sublime, but this is because they have been highly engineered to be this way. The world of fast food is truly the world of artificial food, and the long-range health effects of so many of their ingredients are unknown and have not been fully tested. I would avoid these foods.

3. **Eat foods with no or low amounts of refined sugar.** With sugar, many people look for specific numbers or quantities, which can be an overtly time-consuming and cumbersome process. I simply recommend avoiding foods that are overly sweet to the taste, unless they're a natural product, such as fruit and honey.

---

3 The Food and Drug Administration Modernization Act of 1997 eliminates the requirement of the FDA's premarket approval for most packaging and other substances that come in contact with food and may migrate into it. Instead, the law establishes a process whereby the manufacturer can notify the agency of its intent to use certain food contact substances and, unless the FDA objects within 120 days, the manufacturer may proceed with the marketing of the new product.

4. **I also often recommend low-lactose foods.** The enzyme required to break down lactose begins to decrease in our bodies after early childhood, making digesting large quantities of lactose-containing foods more difficult. Avoiding such foods, such as animal dairy products, can sometimes help relieve symptoms such as abdominal discomfort and pain.

5. **Eat your veggies and fruits!** Your microbiome needs many different types of bacteria to help break down your food. By eating more complex, varied foods, you will help foster this diversity, which is likely to play an important role in improving or decreasing your disease activity.

Frequently Asked Questions

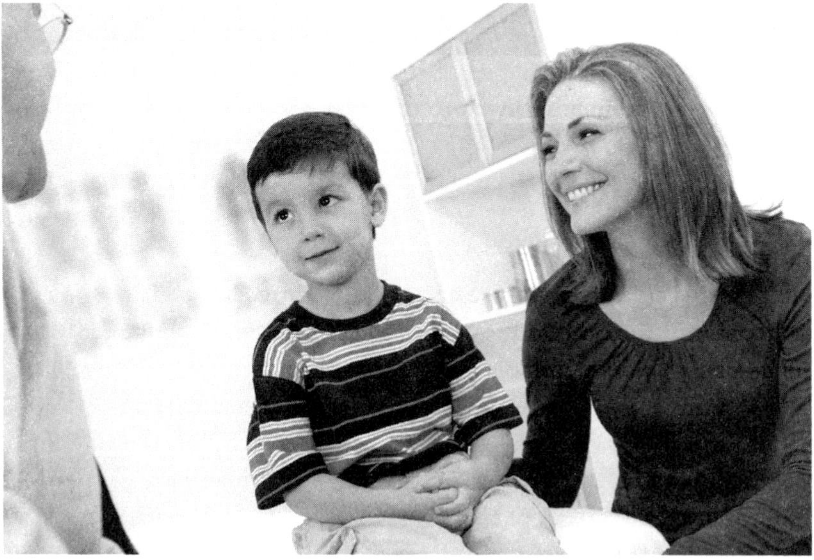

Frequently Asked Questions

Going on—and staying on—the SCD is a major undertaking, but it is a great commitment to better health without the need to depend on medication. But it can be overwhelming, and you may have many questions.

Is the specific carbohydrate diet right for me or my child?

Only you with the help of your healthcare provider can answer this question. Any decision on treatment, whether it is based on medication or diet, needs to balance the therapy's potential success with its possible drawbacks or side effects. When deciding upon a treatment course, important points to consider include the severity of the disease, how complicated the disease is, the potential side effects of the treatment itself, and difficulties in complying with the therapy. See pages 17–30 in "The Specific Carbohydrate Diet: What It Is and If It's Right for You" for more information.

If my child refuses to do the SCD, should I force her do it?

For the specific carbohydrate diet to be successful, everybody needs to be on board! Never force or use excess pressure to make your child use dietary therapy. If your child puts up strong resistance to the SCD and is forced to trial it, chances are it will fail. The goal in dietary therapy is to offer a treatment option that can be used throughout a lifetime. To avoid destroying the chances of your child using dietary therapy later in life by making the experience onerous, simply educate them. And when (or if) they want to consider the SCD, allow it to happen. In short, the SCD has to be a collaborative process between you, your whole family, and your child. See pages 17–30 in "The Specific Carbohydrate Diet: What It Is and If It's Right for You" and pages 31–40 in "Getting on the SCD and Sticking with It" for more information.

Are the medications to treat inflammatory bowel disease bad?

Medications to treat IBD are important to ensure that people with the disease are able to live a healthy, productive, and happy life. Life decisions are rarely black-and-white. The decision to trial dietary therapy can be right for many, but it is not necessarily for everybody. The medications we use to treat IBD are able to reverse the symptoms as well as the associated inflammation. And this is essential! All medications have potential side effects. And these side effects can be scary, especially to a parent of a young child; with that said, significant side effects will occur if a patient can't get into remission. That is why regardless of what treatment option is decided upon—whether diet or medication—the primary goal is not only to get that individual feeling better and doing well but also to get the inflammation under control.

How long does it take to see the effects of the specific carbohydrate diet? And does it work for everyone?

The first part of the question is hard to answer, as the SCD has not been extensively researched. The majority of patients I have seen have had positive results within 2 to 4 weeks. Complete remission of symptoms can take longer—up to 6 to 12 weeks. An important point to make is that if you are not seeing some improvement by 3 to 4 weeks, additional or alternative therapy should be considered; if the symptoms are worsening, the decision to change therapy should be made sooner.

The SCD does not work for everybody. Is important to have close follow-up with your healthcare provider and dietitian to help make sure your child gets the best possible care. If the diet does not work for you or your child, it is imperative to consider alternative or additional therapy as quickly as possible. Childhood is a time of both physical and mental growth. Active disease can compromise both.

If the diet doesn't work is for me or my child, does that mean I should stop doing it and try again later?

The cause of inflammatory bowel disease has two aspects: First, the immune system that is attacking the bowels, and second, the microbiome that is triggering the immune system to attack the bowels. The dietary therapy works on the microbiome and therefore allows the immune system to quiet down. In some cases, the immune system has become so overactive that it may not subside simply by changing the diet. In this scenario, alternative or additional medical therapy should be considered. Once the immune system has quieted down, the SCD may be more effective.

What are some of the pitfalls when starting the SCD?

Prior to starting the SCD, it is important to understand the basics of the diet and to have a strategy of how you are going to make this dietary transition possible. Plan ahead! Make sure you have the time needed as well as support of other family members and friends. Also try to find local and online SCD communities that can support your efforts as well. See pages 31–40 in "Getting on the SCD and Sticking with It" for more information.

Common pitfalls include misaligning the SCD with other alternative therapies. Other dietary therapies such as juicing are counterproductive and counterintuitive to the SCD. Big misconceptions also persist regarding over-the-counter dietary supplements. They are a multibillion dollar industry with little regulatory oversight, meaning that manufacturers aren't required to test their products or even provide proof of how their products affect health. This means that we often don't know the true effects of these therapies. In addition, many studies have shown that often what is labeled on a nutraceutical is not even present in the product. Buyer beware!

Do you recommend taking a multivitamin when on the SCD?

Not necessarily. It depends on the dietary intake of the individual. The SCD, if done correctly, meets complete nutritional needs. In an analysis of patients here at Seattle Children's, the only vitamin intake that rated consistently lower than the recommended daily allowance (RDA) was vitamin D. We therefore routinely supplement with vitamin D. Every individual on the SCD should be seen by a dietitian. The dietician should do a 3-day dietary and nutritional analysis to ensure that an individual is getting enough vitamin and minerals. If your child is not getting enough vitamins and minerals, a daily supplemental multivitamin would be appropriate. See page 29 for more information.

What are the major concerns for families and children starting the SCD?

Eating is not only important to ensuring good health, but it can also be a social experience. We socialize, tell stories, and bond with others over meals. Being on a restrictive diet sometimes gets in the way of this shared experience. For children and adolescents, this can be difficult and it sometimes makes individuals feel excluded or socially awkward. To combat this, one needs to be proactive and make sure that the diet does not get in the way of daily activity.

For sporting events, make sure the right SCD foods are available to give your child that extra boost. Bananas, dried fruit bars, and nut butters can be a good source of energy prior to participating in vigorous sports.

For social outings, movies, and get-togethers, having easily accessible and portable snack foods makes everything easier and less awkward. As with so much in life, being open and talking with other families and friends can make the SCD far simpler. Trying to hide it or going to lengths to not draw attention to it can often make things more stressful and cumbersome. Going on the SCD should mean embracing it and not feeling ashamed about it.

In addition, with IBD there is always concern (whether on dietary therapy or medication) about proper weight gain and growth. Because the SCD restricts a lot of high-calorie foods, weight gain is something we always look out for. The majority of the SCD children we follow gain weight and grow appropriately, but we are always proactively watching our patients' nutritional health. If weight gain is an issue, finding foods that are higher in calories that your child actually likes to eat is imperative.

See pages 17–30 in "The Specific Carbohydrate Diet: What It Is and If It's Right for You" and pages 31–40 in "Getting on the SCD and Sticking with It" for more information.

If my child is doing well on Stage 2 of the SCD (maintenance stage), do I have to add in foods?

There is no need to add in so-called "illegal" foods on the SCD. The SCD itself is a nutritionally balanced diet. We do sometimes add in some illegal foods for some children, because the diet can be too difficult to maintain long-term without additional foods. There is a risk to adding new foods, as this could potentially trigger a flare of symptoms. With that said, for some children we have added rice, oatmeal, cocoa powder, spelt, and potatoes. If you do add foods, make sure it is in a slow, stepwise fashion. Currently, we evaluate for clinical symptoms as well as get baseline laboratory reports (including stool calprotectin tests) prior to starting a new food. We then see how an individual does and recheck the lab results one month after initiating a new food.

Can other family members who don't have IBD go on the SCD?

Yes! Having a supportive family is one of the keys to success in the SCD. Support can be given in many ways, including starting the diet yourself. In many of the families of IBD children that I see in the clinic, the parents do the SCD as well. For them, the SCD has often been a gift in disguise. While their children get better and gain weight, many of the parents (who may be carrying a few extra pounds) have lost significant weight because of the types of foods restricted and allowed on the diet. So feel free to support your child's health as well as your own by starting the SCD. Before starting any diet, it is important to make sure that from a health perspective it would be appropriate for you. Talking with your healthcare provider is key in making these decisions.

What if my child flares (suddenly gets worse) on the diet? Does he need to go on medication?
Flares can occur for both people on medication and on dietary therapy. While the cause of a flare is not always apparent, treating it as quickly as possible is imperative. Most individuals can treat a flare by going back on the earlier stages of the diet. For those with severe symptoms, medication can be appropriate.

What happens if my child breaks the diet?
The main goal of the SCD is to achieve remission, meaning controlling symptoms and normalizing laboratory results. Occasionally eating non-SCD foods may not induce symptoms, but it may increase inflammation. We need both to be consistently in control. Staying true to the diet is essential for its success. If your child needs to break the diet, do it in a systematic way to see if the foods added are turning out to be safely tolerated. We do baseline laboratory testing, including stool calprotectin tests, and then repeat it in a month to make sure no adverse symptoms are appearing and that the child is properly tolerating the food. If gastrointestinal symptoms do occur, returning to the previous SCD should quickly improve them. An inadvertent break in the diet can happen. If it does, don't worry—just maintain a steady course.

What can my child eat when dining out at restaurants?
Dining out can be challenging. Choose plain meats, fish, fresh salads, and steamed vegetables. Avoid eating at chain and fast-food restaurants; high-quality establishments are best. See pages 71–72 in "How To SCD Everyday" for more information.

Does eating organic, non-GMO foods really matter?
Although no direct studies have been done in this area, I do believe that the quality of our food does impact our digestive microbiomes and therefore

influences our disease activity. I recommend high-quality foods that are organic and free of added preservatives, chemicals, and conventional pesticides, as well as meats from animals raised without antibiotics. See pages 21–23 in "The Specific Carbohydrate Diet: What It Is and If It's Right for You" for more information.

Where can I find a complete list of SCD-legal and illegal foods?
I recommend www.breakingtheviciouscycle.info or www.pecanbread.com.

We lapsed on the SCD for a couple of days. Now what do we do?
If there is a lapse in the diet and your child is not experiencing any overt IBD symptoms, restart the SCD at the last stage they were on. If there is a lapse and your child is having symptoms, consider restarting the SCD at the beginning stages.

How can my child handle the social pressure and temptation at school, social situations, and from family and friends to break the diet without appearing rude? He is also sometimes afraid to speak up or advocate for himself, especially in social situations. How can I help?
We live in a time where focused diets are not uncommon. Many people have already heard of gluten-free diets for celiac or elimination diets for food allergies. Most people will not overtly pressure an individual if they know that there are specific foods a person needs to stay away from. The best way to avoid temptation and social pressure is to be open and proud about being on a dietary therapy. Family and friends should understand. And if they don't, be strong and proud, and let them know that "no means no" when it comes to breaking the diet.

Social situations can be hard for many children, with or without having a primary medical issue. The best way for children to learn to advocate for themselves is to ensure that they feel comfortable with their own identities. No magic bullets exist, but there are potential remedies. Children blossom and become stronger individuals when they interact with their peers with IBD.

For instance, the difference I see in individual children before and after going to the Crohn's and Colitis Foundation Camp is remarkable. Getting children involved in IBD-related groups can give them knowledge, confidence, and strength. Through a supportive community, knowledge, and knowing that they are not alone, children are empowered. See pages

17–30 in "The Specific Carbohydrate Diet: What It Is and If It's Right for You" and pages 31–40 in "Getting on the SCD and Sticking with It" for more information.

Besides this book, what resources are available for parents of SCD children?

There are many books, online forums, and websites. These can be helpful, but don't feel you need to read them all. Start with the basics on the Breaking the Vicious Cycle website (www.breakingtheviciouscycle.info), and move on from here. And don't forget to connect with other families who have already traveled on the path of initiating the SCD. SCD families on Facebook can be very helpful in suggesting other resources and how to do the SCD on a daily basis. See pages 80–84 in "SCD and Cooking Resources" for more information.

My child is a super-picky eater. How is he ever going to get proper nutrition between that and the SCD?

The SCD can be hard for individuals if they are super-picky eaters. It's important that your child is not only able to get into remission on the diet, but that they are able to thrive on it both physically and mentally. If your child is a super-picky eater and is limiting their food intake significantly, and all attempts to get your child to eat more does not work, it may be worthwhile considering an alternative therapy. See pages 17–30 in "The Specific Carbohydrate Diet: What It Is and If It's Right for You" and pages 31–40 in "Getting on the SCD and Sticking with It" for more information.

My child is having constipation issues. What should we do about this?

Constipation can occur on the SCD, especially if your child is not drinking enough water. If a child is constipated, I make sure they are drinking enough water (i.e., their urine is clear to a pale yellow color) and are ingesting enough fiber in their diet. If there are no issues with water or diet, I advise drinking prune juice or eating whole prunes with the goal of at least one soft bowel movement once a day to once every other day. See "Constipation" on page 76 for more information.

Why is my child not getting better on the SCD?

There are a number of potential reasons why a child is not getting better on the SCD. The first question is whether illegal foods are getting into the diet inadvertently. I often have a family record a 3-day diet log that quantifies what and how much of each food the child is eating. I'll have them go through this with our dietitian to see if any illegal foods are creeping into the diet.

I also look at any over-the-counter dietary supplements recorded in the log. As I mentioned before, dietary supplements are not regulated, and it is hard to know their true impact on the fecal microbiome.

The second question is if the child is truly being compliant with the diet. If a child is not motivated to be on it, adherence is likely low, and an alternative therapy should be explored.

Finally, it may be that the SCD is just not effective for your child. I've had patients and families who were diligent in assuring that no illegal foods were eaten, and still the diet did not work. In these situations, it's important to move on to another therapy. See pages 17–30 in "The Specific Carbohydrate Diet: What It Is and If It's Right for You" and pages 31–40 in "Getting on the SCD and Sticking with It" for more information.

Is caffeine allowed on the SCD?

Caffeine in the form of coffee and tea is allowed, although it should be in moderation, as caffeine is a stimulant and excessive amounts can cause gastrointestinal problems, including cramping.

Are herbal remedies allowed when one is on the SCD?

Caution should be used when considering additional herbal supplements or other alternative therapies. The impact of such therapies is hard to quantify for patients with inflammatory bowel disease. I have met families where the SCD did not seem to be working effectively, but when other adjunct therapies were removed, the SCD worked. Given the fact that the supplement business is not regulated and that most supplements have not been properly evaluated in IBD, I caution against their use.

Is it possible to eat too much of any one SCD-legal food and have problems?

It is not only possible to eat too much of one SCD legal food, but it is also a common issue for some children. I often see this with sweeter foods such as fruits or fruit bars. These foods can add excess fructose, which causes gas and thus further contributes to abdominal discomfort. If you notice that your child is eating a limited diet, it is worthwhile to meet with your dietitian to discuss strategies to expand their food intake. See pages 78–79 in "Diet Problems" for more information.

How can I support and further the SCD?

Much more needs to be done to understand the impact of nutrition in IBD as well as in other areas of human health and disease. Be a vocal advocate. Talk with your community leaders, your national leaders, the Crohn's and Colitis Foundation of America (CCFA), and local and research gastroenterologists, and tell them that more needs to be done for research in nutrition and IBD (as well as every other autoimmune disorder and cancer!). And support research efforts—through knowledge comes understanding.

The Future of SCD

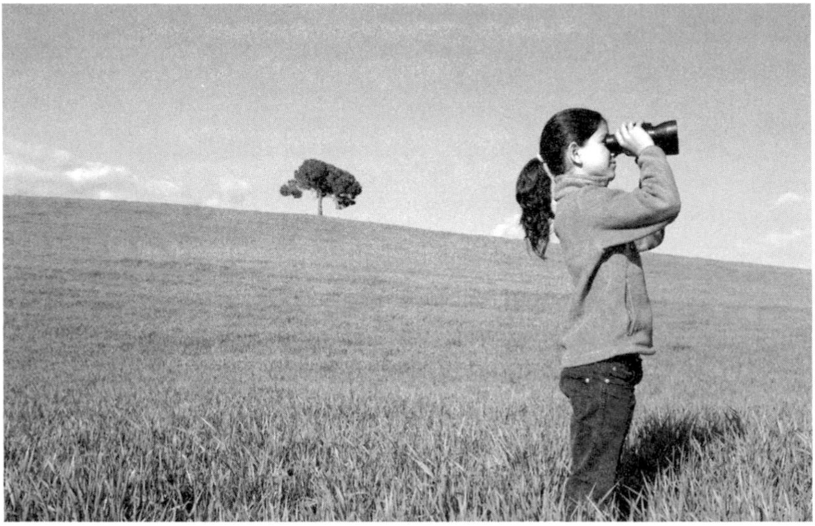

The Future of SCD

At Seattle Children's Hospital, we are committed to making sure that the children we see receive the best care, whether it is based on medication or nutrition. Our research and clinical experience within our IBD center has given us insight into the power of nutrition in IBD. Nutrition in Immune Balance (NIMBAL) therapy is a standardized dietary approach based upon our current understanding of the impact of diet on the microbiome and IBD. This book marks the first steps of integrating dietary therapy into mainstream medical practice for IBD.

Despite our success with dietary interventions in IBD, many questions remain unanswered. What components of the diet are the most important? Why does the diet work for some and not others? Can we predict outcomes based upon an individual's fecal microbiome? These and many other questions still need to be answered.

Research drives medical innovation and will answer these questions. The SCD started because of the insight and research of a physician who saw its dramatic effect on disease. These initial papers written on SCD shaped a generation of healthcare providers who treated celiac disease.

We are now embarking on a new era of research and understanding of the power of diet in IBD. Our research and that of others will continue to ensure that patients who wish to use dietary therapy will have the best information and resources.

We will update this book as research progresses and we garner further knowledge. You can see more information on our research at http://www.seattlechildrens.org/medical-staff/David-L-Suskind/.

For individuals interested in supporting further research in the SCD, nutrition, and IBD, please go to http://giveto.seattlechildrens.org/ibd.

About the Author

David L. Suskind, MD is attending physician at Seattle Childrens Hospital and professor of pediatrics at the University of Washington School of Medicine. An expert in intestinal diseases, Suskind has focused much of his energy into clinical care and research for inflammatory bowel disease.